Reconstructing Bodies

Studies of the Weatherhead East Asian Institute, Columbia University

The Studies of the Weatherhead East Asian Institute of Columbia University were inaugurated in 1962 to bring to a wider public the results of significant new research on modern and contemporary East Asia.

A complete list of titles in this series can be found online at www.columbia.edu/cu/weai/weatherhead-studies.html.

Reconstructing Bodies

Biomedicine, Health, and Nation Building in South Korea since 1945

John P. DiMoia

Stanford University Press
Stanford, California

Stanford University Press
Stanford, California

Printed and bound by CPI Group (UK) Ltd, Croydon, CR0 4YY

Library of Congress Cataloging-in-Publication Data

DiMoia, John Paul, author.
Reconstructing bodies : biomedicine, health, and nation-building in South Korea since 1945 / John P. DiMoia.
pages cm. — (Studies of the Weatherhead East Asian Institute, Columbia University)
Includes bibliographical references and index.
ISBN 978-0-8047-8411-5 (cloth : alk. paper)
1. Medicine—Korea (South)—History—20th century. 2. Public health—Korea (South)—History—20th century. 3. Medical policy—Korea (South)—History—20th century. I. Title. II. Series: Studies of the Weatherhead East Asian Institute, Columbia University.
R627.D56 2013
362.1095195—dc23

2012043939

Typeset by Thompson Type in 10/14 Minion

KOREA KF FOUNDATION 한국국제교류재단 The Korea Foundation has provided financial assistance for the undertaking of this publication project.

Acknowledgments

THIS BOOK HAS ITS ORIGINS in an extended series of conversations dating to the mid- to late 1970s. My father, a biochemist turned child psychiatrist, and my mother, a pediatrician, encouraged my siblings and me to develop an interest in the broader world of medicine, and they frequently hinted at the possibility of bringing up clinical matters if we misbehaved at the table. Although it was years before I figured out that neither of them was particularly clinically oriented, the majority of the details emerging from their imaginative rendering rather than firsthand experience, my fascination with the intersection between tangible, material practice and the human body first developed here. The present volume is therefore dedicated to my parents, who encouraged an inexplicable interest in modern East Asia and the history of medicine through several lengthy periods of living abroad in South Korea and Japan, as well as through the intervening years of graduate school. I would also like to thank my aunt, Sister Helen Marie Raycraft, for providing a model for living abroad.

In addition to my family, I want to thank Princeton University and the Program in History of Science for providing generous funding and an institutional home in the United States and for arranging accommodations while abroad. Columbia University, Seoul National University, and UCLA each deserve mention for hosting me as a visitor at various points (between 2003 and 2006), helping me to negotiate between the diverse worlds of the history of science, the history of medicine, and East Asia. For training in Korean language, in which I continue to learn (and still struggle), I wish to thank Sogang University and Yonsei University. In the course of conducting research, I have been fortunate to receive research and travel funding from the Bentley

Historical Library (University of Michigan), the Harry S Truman Library, the Korea Foundation, the Lyndon B. Johnson Library, the Mellon Foundation (Needham Research Institute at Cambridge), and the National Science Foundation. I should acknowledge additional assistance from the Academy of Korean Studies, the Korea Foundation, Kyujanggak Archive at Seoul National University, the Ministry of Education (Singapore), and the National University of Singapore (NUS), with this last offering me start-up funds.

Various portions of the manuscript have been presented at conferences and workshops over the past several years, and I want to thank audience members for their probing questions, with a list of venues including the American Association for the History of Medicine, the "Asian Biopoleis" series held at NUS, the Association for Asian Studies, the Association for Korean Studies Europe, the British Association for Korean Studies, Chonbuk National University, the 4S Society, the History of Science Society, Johns Hopkins University, KAIST, Nanyang Technological University, Seoul National University, the Society for the History of Technology, Sogang University, SUNY–Binghamton, and the Yonsei-Yongweol Forum. I also want to thank all of my students from modules taught at NUS, including HY2220 (20th Century Korea), HY2251 (From the Wheel to the Web), HY3223 (Science and Technology in the Asia-Pacific), and HY3252 (From Tropical Medicine to Bioscience) for their ambitious ideas and infectious enthusiasm. Special recognition goes out to Ms. Genevieve Wong for inspiring Chapter 6 with an honors thesis proposal that was never written but that provided me with the motivation to take up the subject on my own.

Of course, it is impossible to repay the numerous personal debts incurred during the research and writing process, let alone to name every single mentor or colleague who has been of assistance, but I would like to recognize in particular Charles Armstrong, Ben Elman, Michael Gordin, Marta Hanson, Sungook Hong, Geun-bae Kim, Ock-Joo Kim, Seong-Jun Kim, Tae-ho Kim, Yung-Sik Kim, So-Yeon Leem, Liz Lunbeck, Laurence Monnais, Manyoung Moon, Robert Oppenheim, Yunjae Park, Dong-Won Shin, and Doogab Yi. It was Dr. Elman who radically transformed my original proposal to study the international effects of American psychometrics after 1945 with a simple request: "Pick a language and a country." Thanks to Jee-young Park as well for her generous assistance with McCune-Reischauer romanization. To anyone else I have failed to mention due to space considerations, my thanks goes out to you as well. At NUS, moreover, I would like to single out Ryan Bishop, Greg Clancey, Seung-Joon Lee, and Mun Cheong Yong for providing a supportive space in the Department of History, along with the STS group now based at Tembusu College.

At Stanford University Press, I want to thank Stacy Wagner for encouraging and guiding the project to completion, along with Jessica Walsh, and I must also recognize the National University of Singapore's book grant scheme for providing a partial subvention toward publication. The Korea Foundation also provided a subvention toward the final costs of publication. I also thank the Weatherhead East Asian Institute for its desire to include the book in their series. The STS Cluster at NUS provided additional research funding through the "Asian Biopoleis" grant provided by the Ministry of Education. Two anonymous readers at Stanford provided helpful suggestions for making a sharper, leaner narrative. Thanks to all for helping the end product come to fruition; any errors that remain, whether matters of fact or interpretation, are strictly my own.

Philadelphia-Seoul-Singapore-Tokyo

Contents

Reconstructing Bodies

Once the Guest started spreading, doctors would only visit the rich—in the countryside you couldn't even get hold of a blind medicine man. Consulting a shaman was the best you could do.

—Hwang Sok-yong, *The Guest*

Introduction

Medicine as a Form of "Ordinary Shopping"

IN A SURVEY PUBLISHED IN THE *Yonsei Medical Journal* in 1960, Dr. Jae-Mo Yang (1920–), affiliated with the university and the adjoining Severance Hospital, outlined the steps taken in South Korea toward the refurbishment of the nation's health system since the close of World War II (1945–1960).[1] According to Dr. Yang, a great deal of work remained to be done, and what he found particularly troubling was not so much a problem of material lack as, instead, a series of inadequate measures adopted in addressing large-scale problems. Specifically, he characterized the administrative approach to that date as haphazard in its execution, involving not a long-term view with careful measures taken to reflect local circumstances but instead a number of "temporary and emergency ones."[2] Moreover, the outlook brought with it an almost deliberate denial of the local, with "imported foreign systems . . . followed blindly."[3] Dr. Yang had previously written on the problems of health care specific to Cheju-do, a small island situated off the southeast coast; his latest effort referred to a series of interviews conducted within the city limits of Seoul, with many of these framing remarks holding for the nation by extension.

Seeking to account for the diverse attitudes of his interview subjects, Dr. Yang emphasized the medical pluralism of his South Korean setting, with frequent intersection between the practices of Western-trained doctors and those of herb doctors and healers.[4] He noted that injections were not limited to the doctor's office and were frequently given out at sites such as pharmacies or even at the personal clinics maintained by traditional herb doctors. When pressed, many patients could not distinguish between a hospital per se and a doctor's clinic, nor did they seem to be concerned about the need to maintain any such distinction. Summarizing the collective behavior of his patient cohort, Dr. Yang would conclude that "the attitude toward choosing healers is not distinct from that of ordinary shopping," despite the possible consequences for the patients' health.[5] From Yang's perspective, South Korea needed not only to make significant material improvements to its health system but also to instruct patients about its proper use and, moreover, to justify why such use might be to their advantage.

Less than a decade removed from the experience of the Korean War (1950–1953), South Koreans found medicine—here referring specifically to Western medicine—largely unfamiliar, despite its growing availability. For Dr. Yang, moreover, the conspicuous presence of medical pluralism was not a positive and resulted in categorical confusion, requiring a great deal of sorting out. Based on Dr. Yang's observations, the present work begins with two framing questions: Under what conditions or circumstances is it appropriate to intervene in the body, and how would these conditions come to be redefined in an emerging postcolonial nation founded specifically on the basis of strident anti-Communist ideals?

Reframing Science, Technology, and Medicine in the Cold War: Mobilizing Biomedicine as Technical Aid

On January 20, 1949, U.S. President Harry Truman delivered his inaugural address, a speech that would subsequently be labeled the "Point Four Speech," with this designation referring to a list of aims outlined by Truman with respect to America's goals for sharing its technical expertise. More specifically, President Truman would emphasize the need for a "bold new program for making the benefits of our scientific advances and industrial progress available for the improvement and growth of underdeveloped areas."[6] With this idealistic language, Truman would explicitly link U.S. diplomacy with America's emerging status as a global power in knowledge production, mobilizing the American academy, along with industry, to contribute toward reshaping the ideals and material practices of a world recovering from the war and just beginning to find its way in the heated ideological climate of the early Cold War. The ambitions contained within Truman's language would soon take the form of the Mutual Security Agency (MSA), overseeing a program that would assume control over lingering elements of the Marshall Plan, and one that would rapidly shift the emphasis from postwar recovery to strengthening networks of friendship with partner nations through new forms of scientific and diplomatic exchange.

From 1945 to the outbreak of the Korean War in June 1950, the United States and South Korea had already begun to engage in this new brand of technical exchange, although primarily at the level of ensuring the security and viability of the new nation. Economic exchange, administered through the Economic Cooperation Administration (ECA), provided much-needed support to the government of ROK (Republic of Korea) President Syngman Rhee, assisting with critical infrastructural priorities and basic necessities, rather than offering extensive training programs or opportunities for further education.[7] The loss of electrical power in May 1948, with North Korea effectively denying access to its power grid, would be regarded as among these critical priorities, resulting in the provision of power barges based along the southern coast as a temporary measure, along with a great deal of contingency planning.[8] Similarly, the purchase of fertilizer from the northern zone would also become a problem, meaning that import of these supplies would become the only realistic solution for the time being.[9] In both cases, the emphasis of the exchange lay almost exclusively on the material end, the physical object, with little thought given to the possibility of encouraging initiative or manufacture on the part of South Korea.

The Korean War would bring dramatic change to this relationship and, even more powerfully, for the nature and scope of any future relationship of technical exchange, emphasizing medicine in particular. If South Korea had figured minimally in American foreign policy prior to 1945, it went from a temporary problem area, an uncomfortable postwar occupation (1945–1948) marked by mutual confusion, to a major priority. Within a decade, "Freedom's Frontier"—here referring to South Korea's proximity to the Communist world, adjacent to North Korea, China, and the Soviet Union—would be one of the new labels introduced to present the nation to the world as a showcase of "free world" practice, a model of what was possible with assistance.[10] The diverse forms of American and international aid made available to South Korea would begin as early as late 1950, when it appeared that victory was imminent, with the combined forces of American and United Nations (UN) armies driving north toward the Yalu River. The humanitarian face of this scenario made for an appealing sell, offering to potential donors the possibility of contributing to the reconstruction of a nation unified through a brief conflict.

The human face of the war, presented both during and following the conflict, brought the nation of South Korea into American homes for the first time on a regular basis, with standard images underscoring the difficulties faced by refugees, along with related problems that lay ahead for the lengthy process of rebuilding.[11] In the majority of these accounts, historical context was lacking, and the basic necessities required for subsistence tended to be associated with the contingencies of wartime. Not surprisingly, medical and relief work formed a significant portion of the aid packages that would be sent to South Korea, even during the war, with mobile surgical units providing assistance to UN forces.[12] The relationship between conflict and surgical innovation is well established in the history of medicine, with the exigencies of battlefield surgery frequently requiring improvisation to save a patient's life or to at least make an effort in circumstances where conventional techniques would have proven insufficient.[13] Here then was an opportunity to rebuild a "Korean" medicine and, equally, a chance to learn by working with wounded patients.

Making a "South Korean" Medicine?

If South Korea found that many of its activities were framed by the broad contours of emerging American hegemony and its related ideological project directed against Communism, the new nation nonetheless would take the initiative in remaking its own forms of practice, particularly in education and knowledge-making institutions. Eager to begin anew after thirty-five years of colonialism (1910–1945), as well as an unexpected and deeply problematic period of occupation (1945–1948), South Korea would place a heavy emphasis on access to education, with higher education representing a largely unexplored and experimental forum.[14] For medicine specifically, the factors shaping the conditions for pedagogy were complex, with at least three major sources of tradition contributing to the emergence of newer, hybrid forms of practice. Traditional medicine, or *hanŭihak*, had originated in Chinese practice, with Koreans indigenizing the collecting of plants and herbs for medicinal purposes, making this cumulative body of knowledge effectively Korean by increments over the course of the seventeenth through nineteenth centuries.[15]

At the same time, Western biomedicine (*sŏyang ŭihak*) offered an appealing alternative with its message of intervention and cure, marking a contrast with the overall health and program of maintenance associated with *hanŭihak*. In the Korean context, this medicine derived primarily from two distinct sources: Protestant missionaries who arrived in the late nineteenth century and the Japanese colonial authorities, who brought it as part of their package of enforced modernization, similar to the measures introduced in Japan as part of the Meiji restoration.[16] Although the first of these two sources resulted in a generally positive reception, leading to the construction of hospitals and related facilities, the forms of medical practice brought by the Japanese created a climate of deep ambivalence and unease, especially in the form of policing and quarantine measures.[17] Eager to bring medical modernity to their colony, the Japanese would seek to suppress the legacy of traditional practice, restricting its impact first by eliminating the exam system for court physicians and then by requiring practitioners to be licensed with the colonial authority.[18]

In its basic outlines, the story to be tracked here will follow this narrative, addressing the issue of overlapping forms of medical practice in transition as South Korean doctors, nurses, and practitioners negotiated a move from late-nineteenth-century German models of academic medicine—mediated here through the lens of Japanese colonialism—to some approximation of American and international models of biomedicine in the first two to three decades of independence (1948–1975). Although the South Korean life sciences would not develop until very recently (post-1980), I make deliberate use of the terms *medicine* and *biomedicine* interchangeably, tracking the broad patterns of change from the German research tradition to an independent South Korean research practice.

Within these narrative lines, there would be numerous moments of continuity, as well as rupture, with colonial precedents in the making of a postcolonial medicine by South Korean actors. While recognizing the continuity, my emphasis will rest equally on the side of rupture, a story of the consolidation of new opportunities and professional growth on the part of South Korean biomedical practitioners, resulting in a far more lucrative and culturally powerful form of practice by the late twentieth century. In brief, South Korean practitioners frequently picked up from where Japanese colonial officials had left off and from these diverse elements made a hybrid practice of their own.

If the end result may appear familiar, comprising the elite private clinics of southeastern Seoul, devoted primarily to the aesthetic needs of a wealthy clientele, along with hospital facilities including those of Seoul National University, Severance, and Ajou, the journey to reach this point will prove anything but familiar. In 1945, it was still uncommon for a Korean to visit a doctor trained in Western biomedicine, and indeed this would remain the case for some time, due to the scarcity of Western medical education during much of the preceding period. Encounters with biomedicine, moreover, were fraught with tension, as these experiences tended to carry extremely negative associations from the colonial period, typically involving quarantine or some form of restriction, with much of the enforcement for public health linked to the police bureau.[19] Biomedicine, in short, was very different from the progressive force brought by missionaries and tended to be linked to images of conjoined power and policing, whether that of the colonizer or even of the American occupying forces who arrived in 1945, providing yet another source of ambivalence.

The major task here will be to explain how and why South Koreans would come to make a medicine of their own, with the degree of physical intervention—including common practices such as the physical examination, injection, surgery, and autopsy—tolerated increasingly by the most recent two to three decades (1980 through the present), so much so that the nation has now come to be associated with the practice of plastic and aesthetic surgery. If sites such as Brazil and Thailand surpass South Korea in the number of procedures performed, the ROK has nonetheless earned for itself the nickname "the Republic of Plastic Surgery," and ambitious efforts on the part of the South Korean cosmetics industry, along with the promotion of medical tourism, have begun to affect neighboring parts of Northeast Asia. I will argue that these developments are far from coincidental and intersect closely with the historical development of medical expertise on the part of South Korean practitioners, spreading to the population through a series of aggressive public health campaigns in the 1960s and 1970s, when medicine began to leave the hospital site and the clinic, making its way to nearby urban and rural areas through both public outreach and nation building.

If the experience of visiting a medical facility or clinic was one fraught with tension in 1945, and still very much atypical, the encounter with the South Korean state in the form of family planning (*kajok kyehoek*) would become a familiar encounter by the late 1960s, with clinics available in most urban areas and with mobile vans and mother's clubs reaching to many parts of the rural countryside. Through these resources, the average individual could obtain information about birth control, and South Korean women were encouraged to submit their bodies to a wide range of reproductive technologies. Men were also included within the scheme; they were educated about the use of birth control and, in many cases, encouraged to undergo a vasectomy, assuming that they had already fathered children. Although these efforts were largely state directed, the campaigns cannot be dismissed as entirely top down, as South Koreans, especially women, made the campaigns very much their own, actively shaping distribution of the state's resources as well as the contributions deriving from international partners.

By effectively taking over the family planning program through their eager participation, South Korean women were able to pursue their own agendas and also participated in creating new forms of state-sanctioned nationalism. And if the majority of adults met the state through its family planning programs, children would not be left out, as the public schools served as one of the primary mechanisms for distributing public health care, in this case focusing on the presence of intestinal parasites beginning in the late 1960s. The antiparasite campaigns (*kisaengch'ung pangmyŏl*) used these schoolchildren as part of a nationwide survey beginning in 1969, recognizing that environmental conditions—especially the frequent use of "night soil" as a source of fertilizer, along with lack of access to sources of clean water—had brought parasites into the lives of the majority of South Koreans. This development would be treated not only as an endemic health problem but also as a matter of national pride, an index of comparative development at a time when the nation was undergoing rapid change.

As part of these campaigns, schoolchildren were required to donate a stool sample twice a year, creating the familiar ritual of a queue in front of the teacher's desk, with each child holding a small specimen bag to hand in. As with family planning, not everyone was comfortable with this activity, and there remain numerous accounts of those who would skip school out of embarrassment or of children who submitted a pet's sample, typically that of a dog or cat, in lieu of their own. Historicizing this activity is difficult, as these accounts remain apocryphal, yet we should see the refusal to submit a sample not simply as resistance to the state but equally as reluctance to permit access to one's body. In other words, the changes that came with an aggressive public health were incremental, and not everyone embraced these changes eagerly, even as the ROK state sought to tie both campaigns to an emerging nationalism, fostering a sense of personal responsibility.

Along with the changes to attitudes about the body and gradual acceptance of new forms of intervention would come corresponding changes to the professionalization expected of South Korean health workers. Traditional practitioners would create their own forms of medical pedagogy, based at institutions such as Kyunghee University (1965), bringing a hybrid form of practice into being. Because this reconfigured "traditional" practice would not regain prestige until sometime in the early 1980s, concurrent with rapid economic growth, medical doctors increasingly shifted their training to some approximation of international models by interacting frequently with their foreign colleagues at conferences and by making their proceedings available in other languages, typically English. Moreover, doctors would become less autocratic, sharing their responsibilities with a larger number of support personnel. At the most basic level, South Korean doctors would become increasingly clinically oriented, more "hands on," as they grew more specialized in the forms of care they could offer and as their patient base became much more diverse.

Along with the state's enthusiasm for promoting public health, the medical industry in South Korea would change dramatically with the origins of a national health insurance scheme (1977) and with the subsequent arrival of democratization (1987). The presence of cosmetic/aesthetic surgery in South Korea predates both of these developments and, equally, has numerous precedents in neighboring East Asian countries, with Japan figuring prominently as a source of models, practices, and aesthetic norms. The turn to the aesthetic therefore has less to do with social pathology, as some popular accounts would have it, than with the historical intersection of new professional norms; the increasing economic power of an elite, highly specialized medical community; and, most importantly, the acceptance of and confidence associated with medical intervention as a means to realize and achieve one's desired self-image. Although the state had previously promoted public health to a reluctant population, South Koreans would ultimately make this medicine their own by the mid- to late 1980s, eagerly embracing the possibilities of personal change and self-fashioning.

Mobilizing the Traffic in Bodies

When the process of medical transformation began in the late 1940s and early 1950s, the application of medicine to individuals took place within a particular context, with the political relationship between the United States and its partner nation shaping the exchange as a call to vote with one's feet. In other words, the ideological contrast with neighboring North Korea would rapidly become one in which the movement of large numbers of refugees was a key selling point in the propaganda war. Biomedicine therefore represented an aspect of relief work associated specifically with a conscious choice to move to South Korea and carried with it a comforting set of images, caring for and repairing damaged bodies on arrival. This type of imagery would tend to hold true regardless of whether the type of injury was caused by the effects of chronic disease (such as tuberculosis) or by the effects of war. In nearly all cases, biomedicine stood as a symbolic and material means of transformation at a time when movement away from North Korea connoted an escape from communism and its associated material lack.

These patterns of movement did not mean that there was no resistance to the practice of biomedicine, and in fact, as we shall learn, the negotiation nearly always required an incremental set of adjustments. Moreover, the remaking of a South Korean medicine required a corresponding traffic in bodies: the bodies of refugees and patients to be treated, the migration of South Korean elites abroad for access to higher education, and the resettling of displaced populations. Of these three groups, the relationship between the first and the third populations will dominate the chapters here, as the mass application of biomedicine took place at a time when adoption and out-migration from South Korea were at their highest and, more importantly were most visible to the international community. Organizations such as the Holt adoption agency famously brought South Korean children out of the war zone, placing them most typically with white, Christian families based in the United States.[20]

More recently, scholarship has begun to look into the political context of these patterns of adoption placement, examining the ways in which South Korean children tended to be asked to adapt themselves to a limited vision of American life, especially one associated with the cultural rhythms of white, suburban life.[21] Working with adoption, medicine offered a means of repairing these shattered lives, regardless of whether children and refugees could make their way abroad, as in a limited number of cases, or more commonly, make a space for themselves within a recovering nation. As for this second case, the many patients helped by American and international surgical units during and following the Korean War attested to the cultural and material power of biomedicine, especially its power to transform personal circumstances. Moreover, new foundations such as the American-Korean Foundation (AKF), taking advantage of the charged political climate, provided various forms of assistance, perhaps most conspicuously by bringing rehabilitative medicine and replacement limbs to South Korea through the figures of prominent physicians such as Dr. Howard Rusk, an orthopedic surgeon and advocate of rehabilitative medicine based at New York University.[22]

But the movement of ideas, practices, and images was not unidirectional, and this has to be much more than a story of American ideological and soft power focusing on South Korea during the early stages of the Cold War. In fact, the South Korean government learned quickly how to mobilize many of these same patterns of medical practice, corresponding to the incremental growth of its own community of Western-trained doctors, and members of this group would soon constitute a powerful lobby. In the short term, the ROK government would turn its interest in biomedicine into an ambitious series of public health campaigns, many of these having strong overtones from earlier forms of health practice, and this holds especially true for the intersection with Japanese colonial health practice. For example, the energy devoted to family planning in the mid-1960s bore numerous points of comparison with the practice of two to three decades earlier, as Japan had tried aggressively to promote a modern, progressive vision of "scientific" mothering in its colonies.[23]

The success of the ROK state in building on these continuities, even while repackaging the campaigns in a newer vocabulary, resulted in a form of presentation through which medicine and health would rapidly become national concerns. This is particularly true for the charged period encompassing the second half of the 1960s into the 1970s, corresponding to engagement with the Vietnam War (1965) and the suspension of the constitution by Park Chung Hee (1972). With the national antiparasite campaigns beginning in 1969, it is not difficult to read the desire to eradicate unwanted pests as at least partially informed by ideological concerns. To borrow an analogy from the work of Ruth Rogaski, the desire for a body free of pests, while certainly a desirable goal from the standpoint of public health, would become equally about the construction an ideologically "pure" national polity, seeking a population that would conform to the state's goals.[24]

In the case of both family planning (from 1964 through the early 1980s) and the antiparasite campaigns (from 1969 through the early 1990s), the ROK state would invest heavily in appealing to the nation through biomedicine, creating a comprehensive vision of the family, home, and society. Whether residing in rural or urban circumstances, family planning offered the possibility of greater personal control, limiting the number of children and offering the opportunity for "demographic dividends," economic growth achieved by limiting the size of a birth cohort. As the campaign grew more successful and the range of technologies provided continued to diversify, additional incentives were provided: Men consenting to a vasectomy could receive early release from their reserve military training (*yebigun*), and families could even gain access to a better apartment—receiving a higher placement within the lottery system—if they could demonstrate compliance.[25] Again, although these campaigns might appear to be top down and paternalistic, circumstances on the ground were far more complex, with individuals sometimes negotiating the system to their own advantage.

The arrival of subsequent forms of expertise, referring here to the development of a marketplace for plastic surgery and related forms of bodily enhancement, is thus entirely consistent with the degree of control offered by the public health campaigns of the Park Chung Hee era. Granted, the structural logic would be very different, with leading medical professionals and specialists constituting a powerful interest group setting the terms of the encounter and with individual clients generally embracing a procedure on their own, rather than having it imposed by the state. Regardless, the logic bears many points of comparison, with the patient achieving a desired end through a surgical procedure and with these aims often involving the intersection of economic and personal goals. In this sense, the public health campaigns that would build a strong state helped shape the context for the subsequent emergence of a medical marketplace involving the possibility of personal choice.

Challenging Developmentalism: The "Late" Arrival of National Health Insurance and Neoliberalism

To continue with this last point, South Korean medicine has been characterized by deferral almost since its inception, with the state mobilizing the comforting image of relief to characterize its relationship to the population. At the same time, the state has frequently acknowledged the limited nature of coverage by medical insurance, extending this privilege to incrementally larger numbers of policyholders (1963, 1977, 1989), reflecting the changing demographics of South Korea, along with the need to cater to the electorate with the transition to democracy in 1987. Commentators have often described this broadening of coverage in terms of a temporal scheme, arguing that the provision of health coverage has been "late" in the South Korean developmental context, with the state failing to respond as rapidly as one might expect. However, this characterization assumes that the provision of medical insurance is a "natural" development, one inherent to this setting, and corresponding to specific political and institutional changes.[26]

If we denaturalize the transition to medical insurance, it makes sense to recognize that the deferral of coverage has its roots in a lengthy history of ambivalence, with the state mobilizing the image of medical coverage as one of the benefits deriving from its authority but without the economic will to provide full coverage. This should not be surprising, as South Korea was an extremely poor country until very recently, and the provision of social benefits would place the state in a precarious position, politically and financially. What is surprising is the extent to which the state has successfully avoided having to provide this full coverage, even with the political transformation to democracy and the accompanying status as one of the world's most vibrant economies. In effect, South Korea, like the model of a limited number of Western countries, has placed much of its medical burden on the availability of private health care as an alternative, opting to provide only a baseline form of care to the general public.

This complex social negotiation, in which the state and the population debate their respective roles, does not have to invoke a radical critique of capitalism to recognize how much South Korea has adopted the privatization of biomedicine as one of its primary strategies, especially in the last two decades. The recent emphasis on the language of neoliberalism and its adoption by the Lee Myung-Bak state is worth noting here, as this implies that only recently has South Korea begun to incorporate this logic into its dealings with its citizenry. I disagree strongly, arguing specifically that biomedicine carries with it a lengthy history in which the state has granted increasing powers to elite groups of South Korean medical professionals, essentially allowing them to regulate their own affairs. In turn, the state has asked for the cooperation of these professionals and elites in mobilizing its claims about health care, effectively obscuring the extent of the problem and the relative lack of coverage.

As this argument will be covered in greater detail in Chapter 6, the version here is an abbreviated one. In simple terms, South Korean physicians, doctors, and nurses have opted for even greater specialization and technical expertise in recent years, especially since the Asian financial crisis of 1997–1998, and, in turn, have expected a corresponding degree of light clinical regulation from the government. What this means in practical terms is the growth of the private clinic as a form of care, with a growing number of these privately owned clinics and facilities in Seoul as well as in many other regions. If the medical profession continues to be associated with its traditional image of caregiving and providing relief, it should also be associated with affluence and social power, as the financial benefits have increased within a legal climate that focuses more on public health care.

Ultimately, my interest in approaching the issue of health coverage is not an attempt to provide a prescriptive remedy, nor is it motivated by a fascination with the economics of the South Korean health care system. Rather, I want to emphasize the particular role of specialists and the expertise attributed to these figures as a category, especially within the context of the private hospital, as in the case of the elite clinics of southeastern Seoul, the subject of the final chapter. If the emphasis on the widespread availability of aesthetic treatment in South Korea has attracted much attention, this phenomenon is embedded within a much longer history linked to previous forms of reconstructive medicine in the aftermath of the Korean War, as well as to the professionalization of South Korean medical practitioners. I want to historicize the turn to the aesthetic, arguing that the emphasis on reshaping one's body to reflect certain ideals is actually not new but rather represents a lengthy negotiation in which this power is now granted to the individual, rather than deriving from the state.

The Case Studies: Six Sites

In tracing the major themes that have been laid out here—the incremental transition from German/Japanese academic medicine to American and international models of medicine in an independent, anti-Communist state, the corresponding acceptance of diverse forms of bodily intervention, and the adoption of private models of health care—six individual case studies will provide a narrative framework.

Chapter 1 begins with the period of American military occupation (1945–1948), looking at the various fragments from which a South Korean medical community would be assembled following the close of World War II. *Fragments* is the key word here, as both biomedicine—introduced by missionaries as well as by the Japanese colonial presence—and traditional practice would figure prominently during a period in which no single category of practice dominated. As biomedicine emerged as perhaps most critical to the subsequent construction of an independent South Korea, it is important to recognize the diverse contributing factors, as medicine held deeply ambivalent associations from the colonial period and would continue to do so for some time. For the majority of Koreans, access to a Western-trained doctor was limited, and the figure of the traditional practitioner was much more significant, like that of Mr. Byung Sang-Hun (1902–1989), the individual whose career is detailed here.

Providing further context for the circumstances under which traditional practice would be challenged, Chapter 2 outlines the arrival of USAMGIK (U.S. Military Government in Korea) and, more specifically, the vast medical infrastructure it would convey. Focusing heavily on disease prevention and redefining the Korean peninsula in terms of a regional occupation, the American military would resort to large-scale interventions, including mass inoculation and frequent spraying of DDT to limit the possibilities of epidemic. While disruptive, this approach toward public health would be credited with limiting the impact of a cholera outbreak in summer 1946 and would prove enormously influential in the creation of subsequent South Korean public health policy. That is, the ROK health system was born out of this perceived crisis, a situation soon exacerbated by the beginning of the Korean War, bringing with it disease and devastation.

Chapter 3, the period of the Korean War and its aftermath (1954–1960) coincides with the growing importance of South Korea as a model for international development, bringing American and international actors to visit Seoul for the reconstruction of a number of biomedical sites. The chapter focuses almost exclusively on one of these sites, Seoul National University Hospital, and the collaborative relationship formed with the University of Minnesota, taking the form of the "Minnesota Project" (1954–1962), but it also recognizes that similar rehabilitative efforts were taking place simultaneously at other sites. These would include Severance Hospital and its new relationship with Yonsei University (1957), as well as the National Medical Center (*kungnip ŭiryowŏn*) (1958–1968), the latter a joint project of three Scandinavian nations, with Norway, Sweden, and Denmark coming together to provide aid in the form of a teaching hospital.[27] In all of these cases, the Korean body as an object of biomedical research would be very much at stake, and it was by no means a comfortable and easy transition as the hospital site continued to generate suspicion.

In Chapter 4, the South Korean state begins to take the initiative with public health, coinciding with the arrival of a new Park Chung Hee state in 1961. Prior to this, the most common health issues in the ROK centered around problems of chronic disease—tuberculosis, leprosy, and parasites—and, while these concerns would persist, the state could now mobilize around a revised conception of the family and the possibility of changing reproductive behaviors, aggressively promoting a menu of new technologies and birth control devices, targeting both male and female populations. Although the FP (family planning, or *kajok kyehoek*) campaigns proved successful from a strictly quantitative standpoint, with many "acceptors" encountering agents of the state, a closer look reveals that this idealized encounter was often fraught with tension. In particular, by the late 1960s South Korean women had begun to avoid using the Lippes loop due to its side effects, forcing a change to the birth control pill as the preferred option by 1968.

Overlapping with the birth control campaigns, the national antiparasite campaigns (*kisaengch'ung pangmyŏl*) began with a baseline survey in the late 1960s and as of 1969 required the twice-yearly taking of samples from children. In material terms, this meant thousands of children bringing their stool samples to school in specially provided sample bags and the construction of an accompanying infrastructure to process and analyze these samples on a mass scale. As family planning sought to extend the reach of the state at the local level through government, these new campaigns added the public schools as the next target site for attention, making it nearly impossible to avoid the reach of the state during this period. Scholarly commentators have argued that only the style of military discipline associated with the Park Chung Hee state could have made feasible the successful conduct of these two aggressive campaigns, and indeed, as we shall see, the antiparasite campaigns were also concerned with the international sphere, protecting the health of ROK soldiers abroad (as in Vietnam) through the construction of a South Korean version of tropical medicine.

Chapter 6 takes up the issue of the present-day market for aesthetic and plastic surgery, flourishing in many parts of South Korea through a series of private clinics and highly trained specialists. These developments are not entirely new, however, and follow from the historical trajectory of the preceding period, including a heavy reliance on reconstructive surgery in the aftermath of the Korean War, an increasing acceptance of medical intervention as a means to achieve self-transformation, and a medical system designed to protect and encourage the interests of highly specialized forms of practice. Beginning with a longer East Asian tradition, the chapter takes up the practice of blepharoplasty, or double eyelid surgery, tracing its roots from Meiji Japan to a postwar form of emerging practice in many parts of East and Southeast

Asia. The South Korean form of the surgery thus represents a recent transformation of a practice with a lengthy history, and the specific variations introduced can be historicized in relation to the Korean context.

In the end, the story of medicine in South Korea is about much more than simply biomedicine, and after 1965 the story of a refurbished form of traditional practice, or TKM (traditional Korean medicine), remains an equally fascinating line of inquiry. South Korea, like many of its Asian neighbors (including China and Vietnam), maintains a dual system of practice, permitting choice according to one's preferences. Moreover, North Korea would have to be included in such a larger story, with its own version of traditional practice (*Koryŏ ŭihak*), its initial embrace of socialist models of public health, and its present-day reluctance to rely on international assistance despite a conspicuous need. This work will focus primarily on the South Korean case of biomedicine to illustrate that the series of choices made by the South (from 1945 to the present) were as equally ideological as those made by the North, if ultimately far more successful in the eyes of the world, and also to illustrate that the embrace of biomedical culture, while now seemingly "obvious," was frequently a tentative and quite painful one, characterized by deep ambivalence.

I From Occupation to Nation

1 Medicine and Its Fragments, 1945–1948

Traditional Practitioners and the USAMGIK

In 1944, Andrew Grajdanzev published *Modern Korea*, a comprehensive survey of the peninsula and its social conditions following several decades of Japanese colonial rule; the survey offered a deeply critical take on claims made by colonial authorities.[1] While scholars have speculated a great deal on Gradjanzev's ideological leanings and his personal identity, along with his curious institutional affiliation, the Institute of Pacific Relations (IPR), it is the cumulative statistical portrait presented in his volume that holds the greatest potential for further inquiry: Grajdanzev critiques the very terms on which the colonial apparatus bases its hold, especially the claim of penetrating the Korean countryside, even under difficult wartime conditions. More specifically, questions of land ownership, access to education at all levels, and access to modern forms of medical care represent the major issues to be confronted, with an incisive, almost corrosive skepticism directed at the existing portrait made available through standard sources such as the more optimistic framing offered in *Chosen Sotokofu Tokei Nenpo*, the series of annual reports issued by the governor-general of Korea (GGK) as evidence of its benevolence toward the colony.

Gradjanzev offers an image of conspicuous lack of medicine and health care, with only a small handful of doctors based in urban areas, offering their care almost exclusively to a Japanese clientele, primarily those associated with the colonial state and its settler population. This is not to say that the colonial medical system had no impact on colonial Korea. In fact, the legacy of Japan's medical system during the colonial period has recently become the subject of a great deal of emerging scholarly literature, especially with respect to key issues such as gender, reproduction, and mental health. But the issue here will be framed from a slightly different perspective: Assuming Gradjanzev's terms as a starting point, what were health conditions like for the significant portion of the population not seeking care from a Western-trained physician, regardless of whether Japanese or Korean? What were the available alternatives for this sizable pool of individuals, living outside the major cities and sometimes suspicious of, and seeking to minimize contact with, the colonial state?

Byun Sang-Hun's Postcolonial Encounter

Issued in March of 1947, the license provided to Byun Sang-Hun (1902–1989)—here identified as "S. H. Byun"—the third generation in a family of Korean traditional medical practitioners, certified his right to continue operating his clinic at Yangsan, a small village located a short distance southeast of Taejŏn in the southern half of the Korean peninsula.[2] The accompanying photograph, with the left side masked in shadow, offers a sober portrait of a middle-aged Korean male in Western dress, wearing a dark shirt. The individual in question, born in 1902, had continued the practice handed down by his father and grandfather; the licensing procedure likely carried with it a certain degree of anxiety, as it was not yet clear how American military authorities or the USAMGIK would treat Korean medical practitioners.[3] Certainly Byun was hardly alone in submitting to this procedure, as the reverse side of the same document assigned him the number 853, thereby placing him among a collection of individuals who had already registered with the USAMGIK Bureau of Public Health and Welfare. Within less than two years, this act of registration was recognized by an independent South Korean state, which later mobilized Byun's practice as part of its national story by validating his embrace of the "traditional," even while marginalizing his form of practice.

The location assigned to Mr. Byun's clinic encompassed the township (*myŏn*) of "Yang San," located in the "Yung Dong" (Yŏngdong) district (*kun*) of the "Chung Puk" (Ch'ungbuk) province of Korea, specifying the area in which he would be permitted to practice.[4] Comprising a region occupying the south-central portion of the Korean peninsula, the only province lacking access to the sea, Chungbuk (North Chung) was then, as it is now, primarily a rural area, encompassing low-lying mountains as well as agriculture. The town of Yangsan, located in the southeastern portion of the province, was situated toward the center of the peninsula, placing it close to the border with neighboring Chungnam (South Chung). The geographical specificity of Mr. Byun's site was significant not simply as a matter of administrative record keeping but also because USAMGIK was acutely conscious of the need to account for the geographical distribution of medical personnel—including those trained in Western medicine and Korean traditional medicine—in the aftermath of a series of epidemics the preceding year, including a cholera outbreak.

This spring 1947 survey of "herb medicine" and its associated practitioners was only one in a series of bureaucratic activities conducted over a period of approximately sixty years (1885–1945), devoted to identifying, classifying, and ultimately transforming the practice of Korean traditional medicine, or *hanŭihak*. The arrival of Western missionaries in the late nineteenth century witnessed initial contact between the different medical traditions, with Dr. Horace Allen (1858–1932) winning influence at the Korean court through his ability to treat a variety of ailments.[5] Still later, Japanese colonial authorities (1910–1945) attempted to categorize local practices in terms of their own familiarity with German academic medicine adopted during the Meiji period. Byun Sang-hun had previously undergone a similar registration procedure during Japanese colonial rule on more than one occasion, providing a detailed explanation of his training and activities to secure the right to continue his practice as a *ŭisaeng*, or herb doctor.[6] This latest intervention by American military authorities therefore must be seen in its context, representing another in a series of challenges to the authority of traditional doctors.

At the same time, this activity also needs to be addressed in terms of USAMGIK's larger project during the nearly three-year period of its occupation (September 1945–August 1948), a legacy of the unexpected collapse of Japanese forces in August 1945. Caught off guard by Japan's surrender on August 15, the U.S. Tenth Army did not arrive in Korea until early September, nearly three weeks after the conclusion of combat. Moreover, many of the Civil Affairs personnel accompanying the U.S. Tenth Army had been trained at civil affairs training schools (CATS) designed for the occupation of Japan, meaning that there was a conspicuous lack of expertise regarding the Korean context.[7] In many cases, the practice was to rely on Japanese personnel and bureaucratic procedures until suitable replacements could be found.[8] The request that Mr. Byun register his presence with local authorities may be seen not only as part of an exhaustive survey of trained medical personnel but also as an inventory of social resources as a whole. As the American military hoped to hand over its authority to an independent Korean government, a prospect that was looking increasingly likely by spring 1947, there needed to be a thorough accounting of available facilities and personnel.[9]

This effort to survey local resources was framed in terms of public health concerns that had been raised during previous campaigns in Europe and, much closer to the Korean peninsula, the conquest of various island groups held by Japanese forces.[10] In pragmatic terms, this meant that the major concern—even above the welfare of the Korean population—was that of maintaining the health of American occupying forces. The need to survey encompassed those elements that could potentially contribute to the spread of disease—including the availability of clean water and sanitation facilities, contact with animal populations, and the regulation of refugee movements—and required the presence of American personnel trained to handle such contingencies.[11] Koreans, on the other hand, had a lengthy tradition of relying on traditional practitioners to satisfy the basic requirements of daily health and were not always certain about the value of Western biomedicine, especially as it had been heavily promoted by Japanese public health personnel in conjunction with a variety of public health campaigns.

Unlike other military occupations taking place at about the same time—those in Germany, Japan, and Austria—the occupation of Korea did not require the removal of a particular ideology or political party, but instead, the removal of members of a specific group, Japanese nationals.[12] More specifically, the Korean case involved the replacement of Japanese medical personnel by local trainees so that members of the former group could be repatriated to their home islands. In the course of undertaking this task, however, American soldiers believed that there were not enough Koreans with the requisite training, meaning that Japanese police, professors, teachers, and doctors maintained their positions well into 1946 and sometimes even beyond.[13] In those cases where replacements could be found, new staff members tended to be Koreans who had previously found favor with colonial authorities and who were sometimes viewed as compromised by their peers. With respect to medicine specifically, this claim has been made by Korean scholars, arguing that departing Japanese personnel were replaced by a group of similarly minded Korean physicians.[14]

Contributing to the sense of urgency from the American perspective was the added contingency of disease control, a problem complicated by the movement of new populations on the peninsula, a subject to be taken up in the next chapter.[15] Horace H. Underwood (1890–1951), a senior figure at USAMGIK and member of a prominent missionary family, was among the American missionaries who had returned to Korea to assist with the task of rebuilding. Taking a position with the Education Bureau, Underwood was ideally situated as an observer and wrote numerous reports regarding the problem of refurbishing an education system that had been largely neglected during colonial rule. In emphasizing a general expansion of access to education, Underwood called for not only an increase in the number of educators but also for the training of "doctors, nurses, [and] veterinarians" willing to work in the outlying areas of Korea.[16] In making this appeal, Underwood reinforced the link between two related perceptions, a shortage of medical doctors to serve the local population, as well as the tendency of medical personnel to be concentrated in urban centers.[17] With this appeal, Underwood backed a proposal that would dominate the USAMGIK approach to the problem of maintaining public health, a desire to rely largely on doctors trained in the Western medical tradition. If practitioners such as Mr. Byun merited attention and were represented in the 1947 survey, their skills and expertise were nonetheless considered only marginally effective. Ultimately, Byun Sang-hun's career does not represent one of elision but rather the complicated story of a set of skills that began to adapt and transform in the late nineteenth century, facing a succession of challenges to its authority. The issue of increasingly sophisticated forms of surgical intervention and the emerging problem of disease control—particularly enteric disease such as typhus and cholera—were only two of the claims put forward to question the value of traditional practice, which nonetheless succeeded in reinventing itself, both as an independent approach and as a complement to Western medical practice in the newly formed ROK after 1948.

Far from a static set of traditions handed down from time immemorial, *hanŭihak* underwent numerous changes over a period of more than 300 years—from the late sixteenth century to 1945—selecting diverse elements of Chinese practice and adapting them to meet the needs of the community. To administer this process of knowledge transmission, a set of institutions was established to educate and authorize the training of court physicians, and these sites would continue to function until just prior to the onset of colonial rule. Moreover, many of the elements described in USAMGIK materials—local variations of surgery and inoculation, practices that were perceived as remnants from the past—had actually been introduced in response to the encounter with Western biomedicine in the nineteenth century; thus, *hanŭihak* already represented a hybrid set of practices by mid-twentieth century. Narrating this series of transformations through the collective story of several (male) generations of the Byun family, this chapter outlines briefly the changes taking place within a sinicized Korean culture that would encounter the transforming effects of Japanese colonial rule, only to be followed by an American occupation.[18]

If traditional medicine has not always received its due, moreover, this development needs to be examined not by looking at practitioners in isolation but by looking at the rapid emergence of newer medical institutions that would come to dominate the South Korean scene. Missionary families like the Underwoods provided a means to guide funding and resources from Western donors to local institutions, first during the colonial period and, subsequently, with independence and the Korean War. These resources initially went almost exclusively to promoting the growth of biomedical practice; in particular, Severance Hospital and Seoul National University Hospital would represent two of the most influential institutions in terms of training significant numbers of Korean doctors and nurses, along with subsequently promoting the practice of public health.[19] In choosing to focus on Byun Sang-Hun, this chapter argues specifically that this second story, which has tended to dominate the historiography, remains highly contingent: Biomedicine's appeal lay precisely in its ability to highlight a perceived contrast with *hanŭihak*, the dynamic modern posed against the perceived role of the static past. Cast as part of the latter, Byung Sang-hun would be celebrated as a heroic figure near the end of his life, a bearer of traditional practice through difficult times.

Traditional Korean Medicine and the Appeal of Its Practitioners

Scholars focusing on the role of Korean traditional medicine typically select from among three periods, either late Chosŏn (1876 through 1910), colonial rule (1910 through 1945), or the period of independence following the occupation (from 1948 to the present), marking the beginning of the ROK. While this approach has produced a growing body of literature, especially for the complex negotiation between the first two periods, it has often treated the post-1945 story as one marked primarily by the emergence of large-scale Western biomedicine and assuming traditional practice as a given.[20] In fact, Korean traditional medicine also underwent enormous changes during this period (1945–1965), particularly following the Korean War, when it began to be taught in university degree programs for the first time.[21] This process of accommodation therefore represents an extremely valuable activity in itself, especially as it took place at a time when the ROK was in the process of refashioning its own independent institutions and practices. In this refurbished form, traditional Korean medicine (or TKM) forms a critical component of the South Korean national story.

In arguing for the adoption of this terminology, I am following the practice of recent scholars of China, many of whom have argued that traditional medical practices reorganized under the PRC have to be treated as a distinct field, comprising a set of practices designated under the rubric of traditional Chinese medicine or TCM.[22] For the comparable Korean case, I propose to adopt the label TKM, aiming to encompass the revised forms of practice emerging in late Chosŏn and colonial rule (1876 through 1945) as well as the new university degree programs that appeared in an independent South Korea beginning in about 1965. Moreover, the analogy between the Korean and Chinese cases is a useful one, as the transformation of medical practice was common to the nations of East Asia.[23] Once an elite set of practices catering almost exclusively to the court, TKM, in contrast, became associated with the rural countryside, thereby making it available to a much wider demographic. In contemporary South Korea, the use of herbal remedies and TKM now stands alongside Western biomedicine as a legitimate form of practice, with many Koreans choosing according to their particular ailment.[24]

Reinventing Byun Family Tradition

The use of this new terminology, TKM, goes a long way toward accounting for the positive image of traditional practitioners. Within the Byun family, there is an oral tradition filled with such stories: At his clinic, Byun Sang-hun would periodically receive visits from Japanese soldiers on leave from nearby camps, seeking treatment for a variety of complaints.[25] A number of these ailments—digestive trouble, back pain, and minor diarrhea—were fairly common, typical of those plaguing local residents; in these cases, Mr. Byun felt obligated to assist to the best of his ability.[26] The notion of the practitioner reaching out to the population, even going so far as to assist Japanese soldiers, fits with the popular image of the practitioner as a benevolent caregiver. In a culture where written records were maintained by only a few, however, there was little incentive to record individual transactions in the form of detailed patient records, especially with the onset of the early 1930s and the mobilization for war with China.[27] In placing traditional medicine in dialogue with Western medicine, first under colonial rule and subsequently the USAMGIK, I aim to provide an explanatory context for the process of its transformation—including changes to both the practice and the social role of the practitioner—while relying on official accounts as a baseline.[28]

Previously, under Chosŏn rule (1392–1910), medical practitioners and related personnel—including here a limited range of educated professionals in fields such as mathematics, art, and astronomy—occupied a secure niche within society, a designation broadly characterized as *chungmin*, or the intermediate class. Not as exalted as the elite *yangban*, these individuals nonetheless held a position far more stable than that of the majority, those responsible for furnishing the labor for agricultural production as well as the bulk of tax revenues. Medical practitioners at this time generally served the interests of the *yangban*, with the court physicians selected from among those who successfully passed government-sanctioned exams.[29] In addition, pharmacists, who produced their own herbal remedies, in tandem with others who sold these products in the market, also held an intermediate status, but, again, they were more likely to cater to the needs of the *yangban*.[30]

The intervention of colonial rule rapidly broke down the rigid hierarchy of Chosŏn, introducing a fluidity that would point the way toward a transformation to industrial labor. For the Byun family, too, this represented a radical change in their circumstances: Whereas Byun Seok-hong (1846–1926), senior member of the family and the patriarch, had sought to work at the court in Seoul, his decision to relocate in 1902 coincided with Japanese influence, with his family taking up residence at Yangsan. Opening a clinic, family members would occupy a different social niche, with the majority of their clients now coming from area residents.[31] At the Yangsan site, moreover, they grew their own plants and prepared their own remedies, with relatively minimal interference from Japanese officials. If the family compound and clinic represented a survival strategy, it later raised issues in the aftermath of the war, when USAMGIK officials hoped to generate an accurate count of these practitioners, as well as to determine an appropriate role in terms of providing health care.

To examine Byun Sang-hun from the (American) standpoint of 1947, he appeared as a marker of the past, an anachronism who had somehow survived the colonial period. U.S. Army officials were unlikely to recognize the multiple layers embedded within the family's history: The choice to relocate in 1902 followed key changes to the royal system for educating court physicians, which would have affected the practice of family patriarch, Byun Seok-hong.[32]

Subsequently, his son Byun Yeong-mok (1878–1923) and grandson Byun Sang-hun assisted with establishing the family clinic and practice at Yangsan, creating a very different style of existence, catering to local residents. This newer form of practice lent itself to the creation of a powerful symbol of the rural community with the emergence of an independent South Korea, and Byun Sang-hun indeed benefited with a corresponding rise in status. For the time being, though, USAMGIK regarded him as a means to an end, intending to replace this type of practitioner with biomedicine.

"Government of Translators"

In contrast to neighboring Japan, where the GHQ occupation (1945–1952) and its accompanying goal of "democratization" represented a major postwar priority, the occupation of Korea was poorly organized and, indeed, an afterthought. With a lack of Korean language expertise, USAMGIK had little choice but to function as a "government of translators," relying on Korean assistance where possible. Along with the cooperation of locals, the presence of returning missionary families provided a considerable boost in terms of their accumulated knowledge of the peninsula and its practice. Horace H. Underwood was joined at the Education Bureau by his son, Horace G. Underwood (1917–2004), who assumed a position at the newly formed national university, Seoul National University, beginning in the summer of 1946.[33] For the Underwoods and like-minded families who had lived in Korea since the late nineteenth century—many departing only with the intervention of war in 1941—medical missionary work formed the core of the American project, both in terms of encouraging doctors to visit Korea for Christian mission work and, more important, in terms of establishing new institutions designed to train Korean physicians.[34]

Two of the institutions designed specifically for this purpose, Yŏnhŭi College and Severance Union Hospital, with the former linked directly to the leadership of the Underwood family, produced a significant number of Korean graduates, representing one of the few available sources of higher education during the colonial period.[35] The return of missionary figures, while constituting only a small portion of USAMGIK personnel, led to the resumption of this project, performing education and medical work.[36] Moreover, the placement of the two Underwood men in prominent positions at the Education Bureau meant that they were capable of exerting a powerful influence. While the Bureau did not mobilize the rubric "democratization" explicitly, the policy of reopening schools and mandating enrollment through at least junior high and subsequently high school was clearly designed to promote ease of access. Likewise, the decision to reconfigure a range of facilities to form a national university—while regarded as a controversial decision in the summer of 1946—carried with it a similar set of motives.[37]

The tension between local practice and Western biomedicine typically centered on critical issues of treatment and intervention, requiring practitioners to adapt their practice to reflect the emergence of these challenges. The USAMGIK emphasis on disease prevention, along with the opening of new hospital facilities, was one strongly influenced by the expertise of returning missionary personnel who had already spent significant time in country. In turn, the reaction of traditional doctors to their American counterparts was likewise one shaped by their prior experience, particularly the encounter with the public health system of the Japanese colonial government. It should not be surprising that traditional physicians might hope to avoid calling attention to themselves, even as they continued to serve the needs of the population.

Still, their presence in terms of sheer numbers was actually greater than that of Western-trained physicians in certain regions, a development that did not escape the notice of USAMGIK. For Chun-buk (Ch'ungchŏng-bukto) alone, there were seventy-four Western-trained physicians and forty-eight "limited area" physicians, with these 122 individuals responsible for the care of a population numbering roughly 1,100,000.[38] At the same time, there were also thirty traditional practitioners, with 113 "limited area" practitioners to assist, meaning that this second group slightly exceeded their Western-trained peers in numbers. In terms of practice, USAMGIK officials—especially the Bureau of Public Health and Welfare—recognized that temporary accommodations would have to be made. This group of practitioners not only had a greater knowledge of the local population, but they also were largely free of the stigma associated with public health, a legacy of Japanese colonial rule.

Remaking Korean "Tradition": The Origins of TKM (Early Seventeenth–Late Nineteenth Century)

The origins of TKM predate this mid-twentieth-century story, linking to a series of developments taking place in the late nineteenth century, when Korea experienced contact with several Western nations, along with its own internal political turmoil. As part of the effort to promote reforms, the Taehan Empire (1897–1910) adopted its own licensing system for traditional practitioners.[39]

In part this measure was designed to regulate the increasing number of such practitioners, which included the categories not only of doctors but also of pharmacists and drug-sellers. The measure no doubt represented something of a necessary compromise, as Japanese influence was already on the rise, with the Western missionary presence also playing a prominent role.[40] From an institutional standpoint, the gesture was extremely significant as well, as it represented the interruption of a system that had prevailed for much of the late Chosŏn period, supplying the court with its trained medical personnel. This is the world in which Byun Sang-Hun's grandfather, Byun Seok-Hong, was educated to serve.

Prior to the late nineteenth century, Chosŏn Korea had relied on a system of institutions designed to provide medical care to the court, as well as to prevent the spread of disease to the capital. Chief among these institutions were the Chŏnŭigam (Directorate of Medicine), Naeŭiwŏn (Royal Clinic), and Hyeminsŏ (Capital Medical Clinic).[41] Of these three, the first two bodies provided for the immediate medical needs of the royal family, as well as top officials and their family members. The Hyeminsŏ, in turn, functioned as a form of quarantine within the capital city, offering food, clothing, and shelter to those suffering from illness, thereby decreasing the potential for the spread of disease. *Hwarinsŏ* (suburban medical clinics) were established outside the gates of the capital as well, with these clinics similar in design to the Hyeminsŏ in serving as a form of quarantine. However, medical treatment here was provided free of cost, in contrast to the city, and both Buddhist monks and shaman healers were assigned to work at these facilities to broaden their possible appeal to the local population.[42]

The monitoring of the population in the form of quarantine fits the portrayal of Korean society as highly stratified, with the most important element here resting on the restriction of the movements of those who were ill. Along similar lines, regional medical centers were also created to anticipate the outbreak of epidemics, with an important secondary function being the collection of *materia medica*.[43] Typically these centers would be staffed by a handful of trained personnel, with a Confucian scholar overseeing the activities of a small group of physicians and medical technicians. This arrangement indicates the emphasis still placed on classical learning, and, as Don Baker wryly observes, meant that "Confucian scholars with more expertise in Chinese poetry and ancient Chinese history" frequently dominated the ranks of government medical agencies.[44] Outside the court, moreover, the regulation of medical knowledge was minimal, and practitioners serving the population at large were not subject to the system of exams administered to select court physicians and medical officials.

These specialist exams, which were comparable to the civil service exams required to become an official, resulted in the concentration of medical practice in the hands of a relatively small number of families.[45] Though there was no legal requirement as such, the preference for hereditary ties reinforced the tendency toward the formation of a tightly knit in-group. Moreover, the exam system tended to keep the numbers to a bare minimum, with only 166 examinations held between 1498 and 1894.[46] On these occasions, an estimated 1,500 candidates successfully handled the medical civil service exam, meaning that the average exam period saw only about nine individuals achieve a passing score.[47] Of those who subsequently went on to serve the royal family in a medical capacity, more than half came from a small group of families situated near Seoul, again suggesting that the scope of official medical practice was extremely restricted, while the general population came to rely on alternative forms of practice, including Buddhist healers and shamans.

This two-tiered system of practice, with an elite medical corps basing its practice largely on a careful selection of Chinese texts, prevailed for nearly four centuries.[48] The use of Chinese sources required adaptation to local circumstances, and the codification of a (Korean) canon began in earnest in the fifteenth century with the circulation of numerous anthologies. Of these, probably the most famous was the *Hyangyak chipsŏngbang* (*Great Collection of Native Korean Prescriptions*), a pharmaceutical guidebook completed in 1433, encompassing eighty-five volumes in its entirety.[49] Assembled nearly two centuries later, Hŏ Chun's *Tongŭi Pogam* (*A Treasury of Eastern Medicine*), a compilation appearing in 1613 under government authorization, represented a further refinement of these sources and was much easier to distribute due to its relatively compact size. *Tongŭi Pogam* not only became the most influential text of its time but also continues to influence Korean medical practice today.

Appearing in the midst of a chaotic time after nearly two centuries of stability (from 1392 through the late sixteenth century), *Tongŭi Pogam* followed the Japanese invasions of the Korean peninsula in the 1590s and preceded subsequent Manchu incursions in 1627 and 1636.[50] Although this work, like previous compilations, was intended primarily for the use of physicians, it would have a greater impact in terms of its popularization of medical prescriptions. Portions of the text were published in the form of small pamphlets, which could circulate easily among a population eager for access to medical information. Other authors would continue this trend, and the next two centuries witnessed the publication of information previously available only to a few, a development associated with more frequent outbreak of epidemics on the peninsula, especially smallpox and measles.[51] In practical terms, groups of families also began to form pharmaceutical cooperatives, planting and cultivating plants to ensure that a supply of medicine would be available in times of crisis.

During the seventeenth and eighteenth centuries, the arrival of foreign intervention—here meaning both Westerners and Japanese—had witnessed the incremental indigenization of Chinese textual sources and, more importantly for our story here, an increasingly complex system for the production and distribution of medicines. Pharmaceutical markets, where prescriptions could be purchased, probably appeared sometime in the seventeenth century, with the pharmacist's shop following in the eighteenth century, as private individuals began to consult those skilled in medicine.[52] Government regulation of the new professionals continued to be minimal, but the presence of outsiders introduced change in the nineteenth century. The end of the Chosŏn exam system in 1894, along with the first attempt to regulate medical practice at the popular level, represented a development that came only after both Western and Japanese advocates of biomedicine had made their presence felt. Regardless of the underlying agenda, the call to modernization was a strong one, one to which the Korean government needed to respond.

Regulating by Constructing Categories

In particular, this first effort at establishing a licensing system sought to differentiate among four groups or classes of professional, the first being the official doctors attached to the court, an extremely elite group that we have already discussed.[53] The second, Confucian doctors, were those possessing knowledge of medical practice but who opted not to exercise these skills in a public forum. Private doctors, in contrast, marketed themselves to potential clients, catering to the needs of individual patients. Along with this third group, members of the fourth, drug sellers, also catered to a customer base, supplying the materials used for prescriptions. These last two groups constituted the greatest number of practitioners in late Chosŏn and tended to have the strongest presence outside the cities, practicing in the countryside.[54] Whether it was motivated by concern over unregulated practice or was making a conservative gesture to limit the number of doctors, the government's effort to license practitioners anticipated similar strategies undertaken by the Japanese colonial government only two decades later.

At the same time, the use of Chinese medical practice within a Korean setting would become identified as specifically "Korean" by about the mid-nineteenth century, especially as it came under pressure from external forces. If the licensing system represented an effort to limit, it was equally an effort to preserve, to capture an elusive form of practice that was in danger of disappearing. If the Byun family underwent a decrease in status, it was a temporary one, as their practice reemerged in the aftermath of the Korean War, this time reinvented as a powerful symbol of South Korean nationalism. Even as their practice was clearly a hybrid of Chinese, Korean, and Western medical techniques, this combination held great appeal to clients in a nation seeking legitimacy for its own institutions.

Moreover, in the late nineteenth century, Chosŏn Korea had to respond to the presence of Western missionaries along with a sharp increase in Japanese influence. The scholarship in recent years has attempted to complicate this relationship—offering a more nuanced portrayal of the interaction between missionaries and their Korean counterparts—and there can be little doubt that the court perceived biomedicine as a means to maintain its power.[55] The first effort to establish a system of licenses was therefore not so much a punitive measure as an attempt at consolidation, redefining the diverse categories of local practitioners according to a scheme borrowed largely from the outside. Along these lines, Yeo In-Seok has argued that biomedicine and TKM managed to coexist through much of the period, with the two sets of practice each regarded as capable of making a distinct contribution.[56] This spirit of accommodation ended, however, with the arrival of a licensing scheme.

Emerging Challenges to *Hanŭihak* (1885–1919)

Ŭisaeng *and Licensing Requirements (1913–1914)*

Prior to the advent of formal colonialism, the Japanese presence had been increasing via a series of incremental steps, first with the treaty of Kanghwa-do (1876), followed by military victories over rivals China (1894 to 1895) and Russia (1905).[57] With this power came the corresponding ability to dictate Korea's domestic and international affairs; in particular, the creation of a formal licensing system for traditional practitioners was first announced in late 1913.[58] Before this, individuals seeking to learn these practices typically served alongside a practitioner for a length of time, usually several years, serving an apprenticeship in the process of acquiring their training.[59] The new system could not put an immediate end to this style of training, but it accelerated the process of accounting for the number of such practitioners, a strategy preceding that of USAMGIK by more than three decades. Moreover, the time and effort required to acquire a license raised the stakes for entry into the profession, resulting in a decline in the number of practitioners.

Taking effect as of January 1914, this effort at licensing, or *ŭisaeng kyuch'ik*, was a comprehensive effort to establish a system of rules for all types of medical personnel, encompassing medical doctors and dentists along with traditional practitioners.[60] An earlier set of regulations had been established at the end of the nineteenth century (1894) but had not offered such restrictive terms, particularly as there were not yet many doctors trained in the newer style of Western medicine. In contrast, the new set of rules required that traditional practitioners be at least twenty years of age and, more importantly, be able to document at least two years of prior activity to qualify for a license (or *ŭisaengmyanho*).[61] This last measure probably had the greatest effect in terms of discouraging potential applicants, as it involved a new process of accounting. Still, more than 5,000 individuals chose to register following the implementation of this measure, petitioning to be among those accorded the new status.[62]

The motivations underlying this enthusiastic response were no doubt complex, and to some extent it is possible to regard the new requirements as less stringent than they may at first have appeared. Under these terms, a wide range of related practitioners—including those who merely sold herbal remedies, as well as those who practiced privately without a formal period of study—could be deemed eligible for a license if they could document a two-year period of activity.[63] In addition, the initial procedure called for the granting of hereditary licenses, allowing these individuals to continue their practice, even as this art was expected to wither away. This convention applied only to those who registered in the first year, however, and subsequent applicants would need to reapply every five years for a renewal. In this respect, the change in rules brought unexpected results in the short term, as the number of doctors granted licenses greatly exceeded the expectations of the colonial regime.

Although the campaign to exert control over the domain of traditional practitioners ultimately resulted in a reduction in the number of such individuals over the next two decades, it also elicited a response in the formation of professional societies and organizations. Founding one such group in 1915, traditional doctors sought to achieve recognition by bonding together, creating a set of standards and practices to define their common interests.[64] This particular society sought to organize on a nationwide scale but soon encountered conflicts with competing interests emerging along regional lines.[65] Moreover, the colonial regime was at its most stringent during the first decade (1910–1919) of rule, with little emphasis on the needs of the local community, a situation that changed in the aftermath of the March 1 movement of 1919. This movement, with its call for independence beginning in Seoul, soon resulted in nationwide demonstrations, with Japan suppressing the demonstrators and enacting numerous changes in colonial policy (from 1919 through 1931). A young man at the time, Byun Sang-hun was busy assisting his grandfather and father at the family clinic and received the bulk of his training during these years in the form of observation, while his two seniors treated patients.

Byun Sang-Hun's Apprenticeship (1912–1926)

If it remains challenging to document Byun Sang-hun's education, it was clearly a hybrid form of training, deriving from three distinct sources: the family legacy, with his grandfather's prior role; his formal education at a Japanese school; and the revised "Korean" training he received in the art of TKM.[66] While he received the benefit of his grandfather's experience in the reading of Chinese sources, the responsibilities of running the family clinic simply did not allow sufficient time to replicate the education of his grandfather's youth. Instead, he served an apprenticeship and provided the bulk of the labor at the clinic while observing in his spare time. In the evenings, he received private instruction in the reading of selected Chinese and Korean texts, a labor that was difficult, no doubt, after having worked all day. As his father also had not been able to complete his preparation for the civil service exams, it is likely that the family had learned how to adapt this form of training to the clinic setting.[67]

As the Byun family has retained its library of medical texts, we can outline the broad features of this period of training. Byun Sang-hun was responsible for learning numerous tasks and functions simultaneously, beginning his training in 1912 at the age of ten.[68] Along with daily reading from core texts such as *Tongŭi Pogam*, the sixteenth-century compilation (1598) considered the formative text of *hanŭihak*, he began to learn about the composition and preparation of herbal remedies. Through a combination of daily reading and observation, he also learned about the proper placement of *ch'im*, or needles associated with the practices of acupuncture and moxibustion, although it is unlikely that he would have performed these procedures on his own until reaching his late teens.[69] For the first several years, his major responsibility was to continue with his reading and self-study at night while observing during the day, taking in as much as possible. His major function was to supply the labor needs of the clinic, freeing up his two seniors for the task of patient care and treatment.

In terms of daily routine, Byun Sang-hun typically began early in the morning with a series of household chores, first by assisting with the preparation of herbal treatments—tending the garden, gathering the plant specimens necessary to provide ingredients, grinding the appropriate amounts—to understand their composition. As his two seniors handled the interactions with patients, he had few opportunities for hands-on work, but he needed to watch carefully to prepare for his future. The site for the family clinic, the village of Yangsan, consisted of a family compound and nearby, separate buildings for seeing patients, and, although there was a distinction between these two categories, patients could reside on-site during treatment, frequently sharing their meals with members of the family. This was not a hospital site comparable to a Western facility of the same time so much as a focal point for local village life.

In the course of completing his apprenticeship, Byun came of age at an unusual time, as the Japanese colonial government held a contradictory set of attitudes toward the practice of traditional medicine. For much of this first decade (from 1910 to 1919), Korean medicine was recognized as roughly equivalent to *kampō*, the (Japanese) term for the practice of traditional Chinese medicine through the Meiji period. At least officially, *kampō* was being replaced by the adoption of Western medicine in Japan, and medical personnel viewed their mission in the colony in modernizing terms, or such was the rhetoric of justification. At the same time, traditional practitioners in the countryside were generally left alone—with the exception of the need to register as a bureaucratic formality—and it is likely that Byun's training continued under these adverse conditions. In light of these circumstances, the apocryphal stories concerning visits from Japanese soldiers to the clinic now take on added significance. Japanese military personnel, familiar with *kampō* at home, may have felt comfortable availing themselves of a comparable set of practices in the colonial setting.

The Byun family library still contains editions of texts reprinted during this period—especially Byun Sang-hun's personal copy of *Tongŭi Pogam*, or *Thesaurus of Eastern Medicine*—thereby maintaining a degree of continuity with previous practice. The family version of this text contains numerous handwritten emendations, although the majority of these marginalia probably were composed much later, dating to the late 1970s, near the end of Mr. Byun's life. The compiled notes comprise a personal commentary on the herbal treatments contained therein, reflecting his adaptations to a particular prescription or recommended form of treatment.[70] As we can date the beginning of Byun's personal period of study from family accounts, he first began reading this text, along with others in the family's possession, sometime around 1912 and continued to train intensely through the 1920s. The premature death of his father at an early age in 1923, at forty-five years old, along with the death of his grandfather three years later in 1926, left him to assume his role as head of the household.[71] From this point, responsibility for the clinic was his major task; if he continued to study, it was in the course of following his chosen profession.

Hanŭihak and the Challenge of Imperial Medicine (1926–1945)

While administering to members of his community, Byun Sang-hun did not present a problem to Japanese authorities, as he had registered his presence—doing so for the first time in 1938—and was willing to do so again.[72] The contested space during much of the colonial period centered not on the practice of TKM but instead on the mobilization of new models of biomedicine, as well as the terms under which it could be taught and practiced. As this was a debate conducted largely in terms of a new vocabulary, traditional medicine was beginning to change its lexicon, borrowing many of the terms of competing forms of medicine.[73] Some scholars have even characterized this period—beginning in the late nineteenth century, and continuing through the late 1920s—as one marked by the professionalization of traditional medicine, with doctors first beginning to publish their own newsletters at regular intervals.[74]

The period following the independence demonstrations of March 1919 is generally considered the point at which the style of government in the colony witnessed the greatest change (1919–1931), adopting an approach geared to *bunka seiji*, or "cultural rule." Many Korean civic institutions date to this period, including major newspapers, public facilities, and academic disciplines. It is precisely the link to the colonizer that introduces an element of unease into the discussion even today when scholars examine the origins of these institutions.[75] In terms of traditional medicine, it is helpful to recall that the typical strategy was not one of outright suppression but rather of gradual replacement. With new medical facilities under construction, traditional practitioners needed to demonstrate the viability of their practice, which would have otherwise lost its hold or appeal. New associations of practitioners were formed in an effort to achieve solidarity, and the topic of traditional medicine gained increasing visibility through newspaper articles and editorials.

This activity was undoubtedly influenced by the corresponding visibility of biomedicine, both in its institutional form and as a set of practices. Sponsored by the governor-general and by a variety of different missionary groups, new hospitals were beginning to appear, bringing with them the opportunity to train a new brand of practitioner.[76] At the same time, it was not clear whether these facilities, particularly those sponsored by the state, were actually intended to serve the local community, a set of circumstances that may have unintentionally strengthened the claims of traditional healers. Regardless of whether they were educated at missionary colleges or at nearby Keijo Imperial University (1926–1945), the small group of Korean medical doctors constituted one of the major paradoxes of colonial modernity, representing a regime that mobilized the benefits of new practices to present its message, while clearly restricting access to these practices to an elite group.

Keijo Imperial University (1926–1945) and Peer Institutions

Located in Yŏn'gŏn-dong, a northern district of Seoul, the facilities that would later make up the medical campus of Seoul National University (August 1946) had a lengthy history dating back to the late nineteenth century. With the foundation of the original facility, the Daehan Hospital in 1899, the reforms sponsored by the Korean government appeared to be yielding results.[77] The hospital site was subsequently reorganized under Japanese rule, first in 1916 as a part of a technical school; then, in 1926, it was formally incorporated as the medical campus at Keijo Imperial University. As the sole university recognized in the colony, Keijo held a high degree of prestige, and its graduates received access to the best opportunities and positions. Moreover, from its inception, the university was perceived as a site intended primarily to educate the offspring of elite Japanese officials and businessmen residing in Seoul, rather than an institution providing education to the local population.

The competing hospitals and educational institutions established by missionary groups had to work within the boundaries set by the colonial government, which served both as their competitor and as a means of oversight. Aware of these constraints, the faculty at nearby Severance Union Medical

College chose to define their mission in opposition to their colleagues at Keijo, attempting to provide the local community with Korean physicians, an aim explicitly set forth in the college catalog. Medical education encompassed both the clinical and research traditions, training students "practically and scientifically, so that they may be able to meet the problems of life and disease in Korea."[78] In the interests of conserving its resources, however, the college was forced to limit enrollment to about twenty new students each year. On graduation, although these students had taken many of their classes in Japanese and were trained specifically to work in the colony, a significant number of them took positions elsewhere, including neighboring China and Japan and, occasionally, the United States.

By the late 1920s, administrators at nearby Chosun Christian College were also contemplating a series of curriculum changes designed to respond to the challenge created by the presence of Keijo. A faculty committee convened to consider revisions to the curriculum wrote that "as a special school (*chŏnmun hakkyo*), the fullest attainment of our aims can scarcely be arrived at," given the heavy restrictions imposed.[79] Like other mission schools at this time, the college could not attain full university status and was forced to operate as the equivalent of a two-year college. In the short term, therefore, the committee recommended the creation of two new programs in electrical and chemical engineering, thereby meeting a need for technically trained specialists. A commercial course was another option considered, as it would provide practical training within a relatively short period of time. With these programs, many of the college's graduates were later among the first Koreans to receive graduate degrees in the natural and physical sciences, although they had to travel abroad to do so.[80]

The cautious attitude adopted toward Keijo by these neighboring institutions was not simply due to its prestige but, more important, to its sanction from the colonial government, which permitted the new institution a relatively free hand in pursuing new lines of inquiry while providing superior funding and resources. In the early 1920s, there had been a local movement headed by Yi Sang-jae, a former Chosŏn official, to create a national university.[81] The group collected donations from across the nation, hoping to generate enough funding to undertake construction of a university campus on an independent basis, thereby bypassing the need to appeal for government support. The announcement of the plans for Keijo, however, undercut any momentum that had been generated, leaving the group in disarray. Whether the university's founding was truly intended to accomplish this end remains a subject of debate, but, regardless, the effect on a nationalist drive for higher education was palpable. Moreover, as the sole university recognized prior to 1945, Keijo played a formative role in shaping the academy, particularly in its choices of subject areas.

As a Japanese imperial university, Keijo took a role similar to the one played by its seven sister institutions in the home islands—Tokyo, Kyoto, Tohoku, Kyushu, Hokkaido, Osaka, and Nagoya—doing its part to integrate the colony into the aims and practices of the empire. Although the number of graduates was comparatively small—with the corresponding number of Korean or *Chosŏnin* graduates even smaller—their influence would be significant in terms of social impact. The figures for the entering medical class in 1926 support this impression of a university designed primarily with a Japanese population in mind, as there were fifty-two entering Japanese students, along with fourteen Koreans.[82] For the period from 1926 through 1938 cumulatively, the aggregate numbers would depart only slightly from this ratio of three to one, with 2,413 Japanese (74 percent) and 868 Koreans (26 percent) enrolling. Comparable figures at the law school and dental schools were slightly better, with entering Korean students reaching as high as 40 percent in some years.[83] If these numbers are valuable in highlighting the skewed character of colonial education, they also emphasize the potential results to which this style of education might lead.

From the standpoint of its curriculum as well, the Medical School at Keijo reflected a high degree of continuity with its peer institutions in Japan, following a program similar to that adopted during the Meiji period. A four-year program, the medical course was based heavily on attendance at lectures, with anatomy representing its core.[84] Lengthy periods of observation in the anatomy hall did not, however, provide for a great deal of hands-on experience, and the practice of dissection was probably not as common as in comparable American or Western European medical schools. In this sense, Keijo graduates tended to be well trained in the elements of the research tradition but often did not acquire their clinical experience until after graduation, when engaged in their own practice.[85] In terms of their social status, Keijo graduates—regardless of whether Japanese or Korean—were trained to function as elites and were more likely to take positions treating Japanese residents of the colony in an urban setting.

Finally, the medical facilities at Keijo played a critical role in the creation of social policy regarding research into the production of new pharmaceuticals.[86] Although this particular story begins somewhat late in the 1930s, it would have an impact on the conduct of the war, as well as on subsequent USAMGIK policy regarding medical supplies. Specifically, war with China in the 1930s brought difficult circumstances, with medical personnel and resources in particularly high demand. While traditional physicians remained marginal as individuals, their practice became of interest to Japanese military authorities in terms of providing new applications. War with China had already created shortages, and the military was seeking any alternative drugs and therapies that might be used in the field. Beginning in 1938, a research institute was established at Keijo devoted to the study of traditional pharmacopoeia. Researchers at the institute looked specifically to the cultivation of plants and the preparation of prescriptions, recognizing that alternative therapies might yield results. In this sense, traditional medicine again filled a gap where practitioners of Western medicine had not yet ventured.

Byun Sang-hun and the Colonial (1926–1945)

For Byun Sang-hun, the latter part of the 1920s and the early 1930s were busy times marked by more frequent contact with officials from the police bureau.[87] Despite the marginal role attributed to traditional practitioners, they often assumed the burden of providing basic health care to the population, particularly in rural areas. The apocryphal stories cited previously concerning visits from Japanese soldiers take on significance in this context, as there were certainly not enough doctors in the colony to treat Japanese residents satisfactorily, let alone the much larger population of Korean residents. If having to document his practice on several different occasions forced Mr. Byun to adopt an attitude of discretion, it also underscores a growing interest on the part of the Japanese. Rather than simply eliminate this category of practice, colonial officials chose to study and evaluate it exhaustively, looking for elements worth developing further.

In the 1947 letter submitted to his local government, Byun furnished a detailed resumé or *iryŏksŏ* for this period, accounting for his activities to date (from 1902 to 1947).[88] This document indicates that, perhaps contrary to expectations, Byun's involvement in local affairs actually required a good deal of contact with local officials beginning in the 1930s, although his motives—whether driven by a desire to participate actively or simply out of instinct for survival—remain a subject for speculation. In either case, Byun renewed his license to practice on several different occasions—following his 1938 registration, doing so again in 1941 and 1944—as the colonial policy of documenting traditional medicine now granted these privileges for only short intervals.[89] The last of these occasions was in August 1944, indicating that the bureaucratic apparatus remained functioning throughout the war. Moreover, Japan had begun to shift portions of its industrial production to Korea as American bombers reached the home islands, and it is possible that effects of this activity reached the countryside as well.[90]

Also of interest is a reference to a meeting of traditional practitioners held in late July 1943, a gathering that lasted six days.[91] The meeting appears to have been organized with the cooperation of local government officials, suggesting that its purpose was not simply the sharing of knowledge among local practitioners but that the meeting perhaps held a pedagogical intent. An undated reference to a subsequent workshop also appears on the same document, an event that probably took place sometime in 1944.[92] Together these activities suggest that the participation of *ŭisaeng* needs to be reexamined, certainly in terms of the extent to which they were enrolled in the affairs of the colonial authorities. For now, the most likely interpretation remains one with motives comparable to the institute for pharmaceuticals at Keijo organized in 1938. As traditional doctors held the trust of the population, it is feasible that the government hoped to learn from them and perhaps mobilize their consent under the circumstances of wartime.

Certainly the shortage of trained medical doctors represented an obvious target for change, and one of the major steps in the direction of a new policy involved the implementation of public health measures, with sanitation and water carefully monitored. From the standpoint of the colonial bureaucracy, however, the responsibility for carrying out specific measures of public health enforcement typically fell under the jurisdiction of the police, with doctors directly reporting any outbreak of disease. Under these circumstances, the police would come to establish conditions for a quarantine if necessary, taking with them those patients requiring further treatment. Similarly, when preventive measures such as inoculation were offered, a temporary clinic would be set up, appealing to the local population to receive the inoculation. These measures, framed within a public health regime, would translate into anxiety for Korean villagers, who resented the intrusion into their daily lives. If inoculation carried with it a negative connotation, moreover, this negative association only increased as time went on. This style of practice also brought local practitioners into more frequent contact with local officials.

Maintaining Continuity after 1945?

The arrival of USAMGIK in September 1945 brought not a radical break with this dynamic of policing but, instead, a surprising degree of continuity in the form of another governing regime that took an ambivalent stance toward traditional practitioners. Specifically, the survey project that captured the encounter with Mr. Byun in March of 1947 produced a report known as the "Smith Report," a document attempting a comprehensive portrait of medical resources and health conditions in the southern half of the Korean peninsula.[93] Named after the senior American official in charge, the report reflected the cumulative experience of the American military in Korea to date (September 1945 through March 1947), as well as its previous experience accumulated in Pacific island campaigns, along with the American encounter with the Philippines. Much more than simply a survey of practitioners, the ambitious report would attempt an overhaul of public health in general; in this respect, it remained enormously influential for the subsequent formation of a South Korean public health, even while prepared almost exclusively from the perspective of external actors.

An "on the ground" portrait of health conditions in early 1947, the Smith report offered a largely pessimistic view with respect to the available numbers of Western-trained personnel, underscoring the need to increase their numbers. At the same time, the comparable figures for "herb doctors," the broad category assigned to traditional practitioners, indicated that the diverse forms of Korean practice were still very much alive in the aftermath of colonialism, even if their numbers had experienced a decline during the preceding two to three decades. If Western-trained personnel outnumbered traditional practitioners by a significant margin overall—with a total figure of 4,303 to slightly more than 1,600, a ratio of roughly 2.7 to 1—their impact was highly selective, contingent on geographical distribution.[94] In particular, the greater concentrations of traditional practitioners within specific provinces—here referring not only to Chungnam and Chungbuk but also to Kyŏngbuk and Kyŏngnam—meant that the south-central portion of the peninsula, along with the southeast, would have a very different approach to health care.[95]

In the short term, the American military would adopt an approach that was later taken up by successive South Korean governments, making every attempt to contribute to the building of a biomedical infrastructure, that is, a system based primarily on Western-trained personnel. Even as USAMGIK sought to establish its hold over the limited supply of medicines and medical resources at its disposal, it also aimed to transfer these valued resources to Korean hands with the transfer of power to civilian authority expected in 1948. For medical pedagogy, this meant the reopening of hospitals and medical schools, a strategy that introduced controversy when students and faculty at the new Seoul National University sought to challenge American military authority over its operation of a Korean facility. For medical personnel, this period meant new opportunities, with the chance to study abroad in the United States coming to a fortunate few during the years from 1946 through 1950. Previously, Korean elites had been able to study in the region—typically either Japan or China—but the numbers traveling any further than this for higher education had been extremely small.

For traditional practitioners like Mr. Byun, the immediate future held uncertainty, as the USAMGIK had permitted him to continue his practice but without providing a clear indication of what would lie ahead. Characterizing his practice as that of a "limited area herb doctor," the 1947 survey had distinguished Mr. Byun from a comparable group of licensed practitioners, those who could document their practice in an official capacity. Not only did this move constrain Byun in terms of the scope of his practice, but this labeling also pointed to a trend that would come with an independent South Korea, a desire to reform and revise the practice of traditional practitioners. The ensuing two decades (from 1945 through 1965) would witness a decline in traditional practice, even while it was celebrated as a core part of the national culture. Only when traditional doctors aligned their practice with a heavy component of Western medical pedagogy in the course of training would they begin to regain their status as a professional group. In effect, they had to learn to operate in terms of the vocabulary and models of Western medicine.

For Mr. Byun, self-trained at a rural clinic, these new programs offering TKM pedagogy lay beyond the scope of his practice. Well into middle age, he had neither the time nor the funds necessary to retrain. Like many others of his generation, he found himself constrained by a rapidly changing South Korea, one that celebrated his practice, even while treating it with ambivalence from both a legal and medical standpoint. As evidence of the former claim, Mr. Byun was awarded a certificate of thanks by the ROK government in 1958, marking the tenth anniversary of independence.[96] The language of the document specifically cited his work on behalf of the nation, even mobilizing anticommunist rhetoric to bring his practice within the national project. At the same time, his style of practice was subject to increasing scrutiny with the introduction of new laws to regulate medical practice.[97] In contrast, his grandson, Byun Kil-won, earned a medical degree with dual training in traditional and Western practice at Wonkwang University in 1984.

If this chapter has briefly sketched the outlines of a particular tradition, TKM, and its placement within the creation of a new national narrative after 1948, it has accomplished only the first part of its task in tracing the difficult circumstances for individual practitioners. Under a succession of governments—the Chosŏn state, followed by Japanese colonial rule, and, finally, American military rule—Korean practitioners moved from a limited elite group associated primarily with the court to a group more typically associated with maintaining the basics of health care, especially in rural areas. With Mr. Byun as our example, it is not difficult to see that these individuals were celebrated by the new South Korean state in a symbolic fashion, even as its priorities lay primarily with developing a different kind of health system. This second issue constitutes the remaining part of our task: Under what circumstances would the ROK government and its partners devote the bulk of resources to biomedicine?

Part of the answer to this question has already been hinted at here, linking the mission of USAMGIK with that of prior American missionary activity dating back to the late nineteenth century. Even with the negative images generated by the colonial public health system, the appeal of biomedicine lay in its egalitarian potential, offering a message of transformation and rapid improvement to a new nation. Moreover, the message emphasized during the colonial period was frequently one of a practice denied or left unfulfilled, making it even more appealing in the aftermath of colonial rule. This was certainly the case for education, and the eagerness with which Koreans would embrace the opening of public schools has been well documented in Michael Seth's *Education Fever.* For medicine, the case proved more complicated, as the associations created through prior encounters were far more complex, creating a deep ambivalence. In particular, the style of policing associated with public health and quarantine from the colonial period lingered in the minds of many Koreans, who had to sort through their reactions to such an encounter.

But from a pragmatic standpoint, the answer lay in the ability of biomedicine to provide coverage in multiple ways, satisfying a number of the necessary criteria for a site undergoing transition. Even as the fate of the peninsula was very much in doubt during the period from 1945 through 1948, the beginnings of an independent military date to late 1945; with this move would come public health, offering at least one candidate for the earliest signs of a specifically *South Korean* public health. In addition, the southern half of the peninsula would serve as a site for migration for much of the early postwar period, with Japanese forces and civilian personnel traveling from their wartime assignments to Korean port cities for repatriation. In turn, the new occupation regime would ask ethnic Koreans to "return" to Korea, meaning that a number of port cities would witness the simultaneous departure and arrival of large numbers of migrants, creating ideal conditions for the possible spread of disease.

2 Mobilizing New Models of Public Health and Medicine, 1945–1948

Disease and Division (September 1945–March 1946): Diverse Responses to a Crisis?

With the close of war comes movement. The conclusion of World War II in the Pacific brought enormous logistical problems, many of them centered on the Korean peninsula, where Japan's declaration of surrender on August 15 registered as premature, a product of the frenzied negotiations following the dropping of the atomic bomb on Hiroshima and Nagasaki less than ten days previously. Recent historiography has only just begun to look at the impact of rendering unfamiliar this narrative closure of the war on August 15 as "natural," looking instead at related issues such as the American capacity to produce and convey additional atomic devices from Tinian Island to the home islands of Japan.[1] Had Japan decided to continue its war effort, the scenario we know might have been quite different, and this holds true not only for the abrupt close of the war as measured in military and technological terms but equally for its effects on northeast Asia in terms of the partition and division of the Korean peninsula. Much of the planning for the Korean context, which took place within the framework of a joint occupation of Japan (see the accompanying map), pertained to issues of providing for subsistence and maintaining order, transferring authority from Japanese forces to a set of occupying forces.[2]

If the story of Soviet and American forces agreeing to meet at the 38th parallel has been told elsewhere, a theme that remains largely unexplored is the material and logistical implications of this decision for public health and medicine, with the movement of bodies across the peninsula placing an

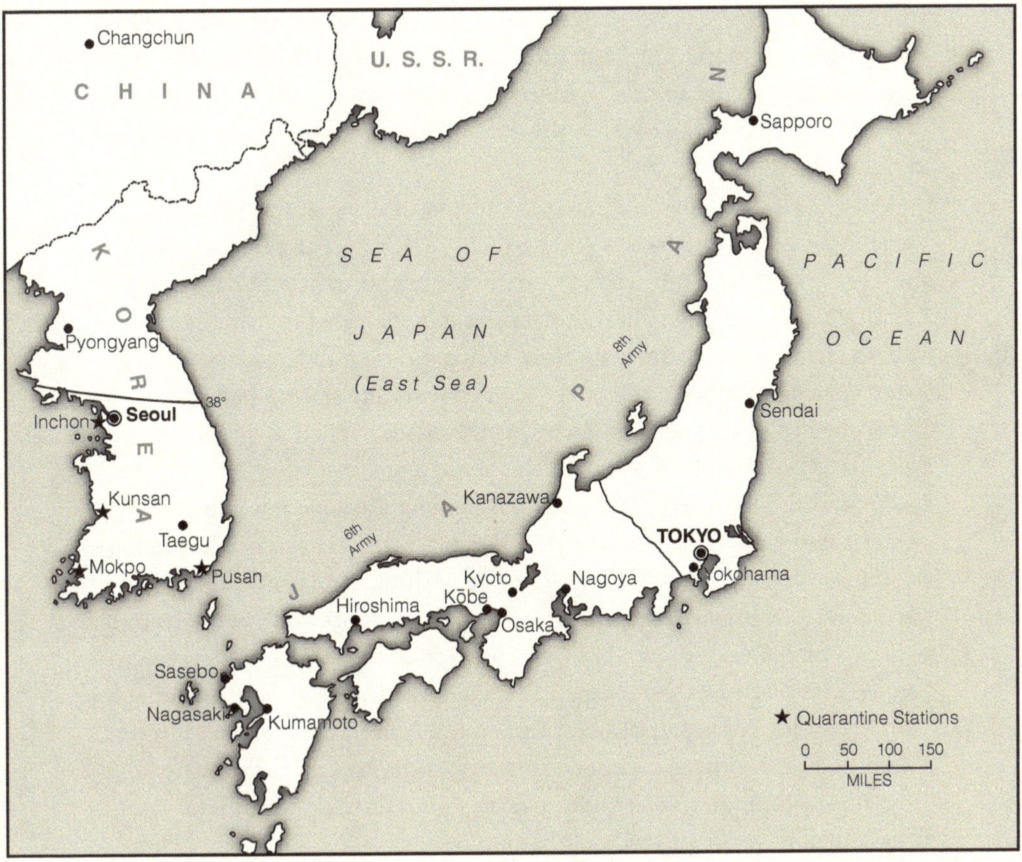

Korean ports mobilized as a form of quarantine in anticipation of the postwar repatriation scheme.

SOURCE: Turner, "Chapter XVIII: Japan and Korea," 1976, p. 693, Map 23.

enormous strain on the limited resources available. The confusion created by an imperial Japanese system that would mobilize a diverse range of peoples in its war effort—Chinese of various ethnic groups, Koreans, and Taiwanese, among other subject populations—would in turn be addressed through an ambitious scheme of postwar repatriation that would seek to return each of these individuals to a designated "home" base.[3] Leaving aside the obvious issues this model raises for ethnic categorization and classification, the joint occupations of Japan (1945–1952) and the Korean peninsula (1945–1948), along with the accompanying scheme for postwar repatriation, would present a significant problem in terms of the increased potential for the spread of disease. A weak colonial infrastructure, allowed to languish during the latter stages of the war, would meet with complications as soon as Japanese forces began to return from all parts of Northeast Asia to southern Korean port cities such as Pusan.[4]

With the intent of minimizing the spread of disease, the American occupying forces, taking the form of the USAMGIK (U.S. Military Government in Korea, or *Mikunjŏng*), arrived in early September 1945 and began implementing a series of public health measures to anticipate problems associated with the movement of large numbers of refugees and military personnel.[5] The major concern at the outset was not the welfare of the Korean population but rather the health of American forces, as was made explicit in a report issued from the port city of Pusan, with the anonymous author prioritizing "the health and sanitation of our own troops among a people not habituated to western standards of cleanliness."[6] In keeping with this sentiment, the four port cities situated toward the southern end of the Korean peninsula—Inchon (in the west), Kunsan (in the west), Mokpo (in the southwest), and Pusan (in the southeast), ranging from the west coast to the east—would be designated as quarantine stations, established to handle the expected flow of traffic in two directions. The repatriation of Japanese personnel, civilian and military, would be matched by a corresponding flow of returning Koreans, freed up from the coal mines of Hokkaido, a variety of industrial jobs in Kansai, and from military service throughout the empire.

According to this idealized scheme, two flows of bodies could be accommodated within a single processing center based at a major port such as Pusan (see the photo on page 49), with long lines of those wishing to enter carefully distinguished from those to be sent home. The two factors of greatest interest here were the quantities of goods to be carried by those departing, as American forces were concerned about the issue of Japan's responsibility for war damages, and the critical question of disease control, with legitimate concerns emerging over the possibility of a major outbreak, such as the influenza epidemic that had followed World War I.[7] The report covering the first three months of the repatriation process taking place at Pusan (September through November 1945) is replete with this second type of image, obsessively noting the presence of "myriad flies and mosquitoes that fed on many years' accumulation of filth, [and] menaced the health and morale of the processing troops."[8] In what became a familiar ritual, individuals traveling in either

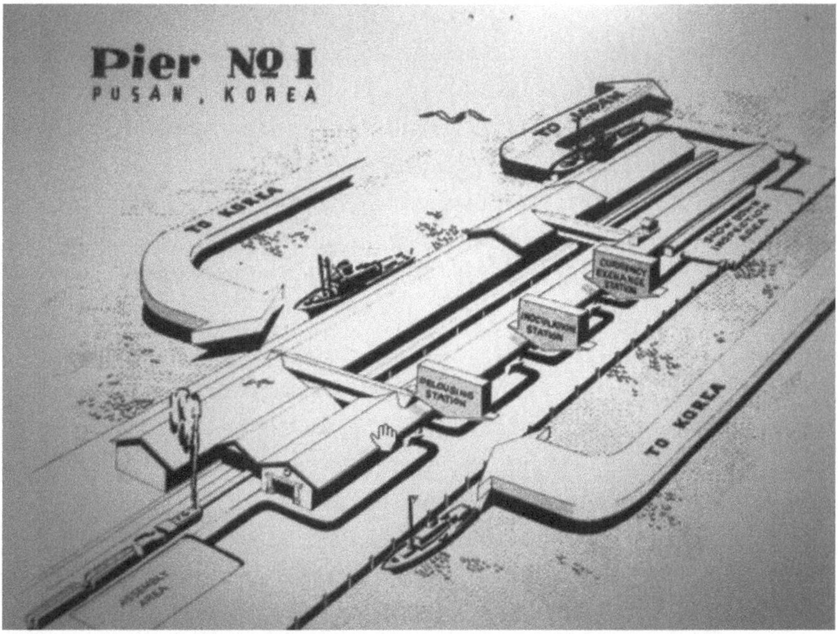

Processing and decontamination center at the port city of Pusan, fall 1945 (September through November), with separate lines maintained for refugees incoming to Korea (located to the left and right), and the outgoing population (center) returning to Japan. Featured at the center are the three checkpoints: the delousing, inoculation, and currency exchange stations.

SOURCE: *History of Evacuation and Repatriation through the Port of Pusan, Korea*, September 28, 1945–November 15, 1945, p. 4.

direction found themselves subject to a thorough cleansing and inspection regime, with inoculations administered in many cases (primarily for smallpox and typhus) and, more typically, all parties receiving a thorough dusting with DDT powder or spray to take care of any "traveling" pests.[9] In setting its quarantine regime, USAMGIK consulted with Japanese experts on enteric disease, such as Dr. Shiga Kiyoshi (1871–1957), perhaps best known for identifying the agent responsible for dysentery and previously associated with Keijo Imperial University.

Prior Sources of Knowledge: Preparing for the Occupation

From the administrative perspective of USAMGIK, with its Public Health and Social Welfare division headed by Dr. William R. Willard (1908–), these cleansing measures were deemed necessary to ensure a baseline of safety, given the enormous amount of movement that would be taking place.[10] If the quarantine regime at Pusan and throughout the southern half of Korea was not designed with the peninsula specifically in mind, it was nonetheless the product of a great deal of forethought.[11] The American military had been planning for projected postwar occupations from as early as mid-1942 and had mobilized its expertise by assembling a number of civil affairs training schools (CATS) based at major universities, including Yale University, providing instruction in language and area studies.[12] The decision to transfer members of the U.S. Tenth Army from Okinawa to Korea, taking the lead in the occupation, was fairly straightforward, given the relative proximity and the need to ensure a smooth and rapid transfer of authority.[13] As with the repatriation process, the focus emphasized large-scale bureaucratic and quantitative processes, confident that emerging problems could be handled as the Americans adjusted to their new circumstances.

As the face of USAMGIK's Bureau of Health and Social Welfare, Dr. Willard, a graduate of the Yale School of Public Health, supported the policies of the occupation by providing a convincing set of rationales for his actions.[14] At least publicly, he did not question an occupation marked by numerous logistical concerns, given very little time to prepare for the move to the Korean context and with a corresponding lack of knowledge about what to expect in terms of available resources. Traces of these tensions later appeared in his published writings, but perhaps the most revealing aspect of Willard's experiences would be the influence of his Korean stint on his subsequent choice of a career path.[15] An expert in promoting public health at locations with a marked scarcity of resources, Willard later designed, implemented, and ran two very successful rural health programs in the southern United States, first at the University of Kentucky and then later at the University of Alabama, making a considerable reputation for himself as a seminal figure in medical sociology.[16] This is getting ahead of our story, however; the situation in the fall of 1945 approximated a crisis, with a need to establish a list of medical priorities amid a confusing set of circumstances.

Along with a handful of colleagues, Dr. Willard was one of the few American medical professionals to receive training for a broad conception of the contingencies expected in a military occupation—with his future posting left unspecified—as well as for public health, more specifically. Following his graduate training at Yale, Willard was serving with the U.S. Public Health Service (USPHS) when called on to perform military service as an officer. If his training at CATS (Yale) failed to touch on the conditions of the Korean peninsula specifically, it did cover a wide range of contexts, emphasizing knowledge acquired during the recent series of island campaigns conducted during the course of war with Japan from 1942 to 1945.[17] Similarly, the coursework at Yale provided breadth of coverage, taking the form of an intensive series of lectures delivered by specialists and overseen by Dr. C. E. A. Winslow (1877–1957), one of the major figures in American public health during the first half of the twentieth century.

Members of the Yale faculty constituted the single largest group of experts contributing to the CATS curriculum, but they by no means represented the only voice within the program, with a range of organizations, both civilian and military, contributing in the form of specialized lectures and course materials. Other participants in the program included members of the Surgeon General's Office and the Civil Affairs Division, along with select individuals drawn from the Treasury, War, and Navy Departments. Given this diversity, the CATS program was designed to combine the highest levels of expertise of those in the field of American public health, augmented with the field experience of those involved directly in the conduct of the war. If the presumptive aim was ultimately Japan, the training was nonetheless regarded as applicable to a range of contexts, sufficiently flexible given time to improvise and sufficient quantities of materials.

Once on the ground, USAMGIK found itself highly skeptical of the Japanese colonial health regime, yet equally dependent on its personnel in the short term, largely because of a severe lack of language skills and country specific expertise.[18] In its stance toward public health, the Tenth Army invoked numerous practices with echoes of the colonial regime, with the repatriation process—especially the twin acts of inoculation and dusting with DDT powder—bringing up unfortunate reminders of earlier forms of quarantine.[19] As the previous chapter has detailed, it was by no means a "natural" matter for a Korean to consult with a Western-trained physician in 1945, nor did it become a matter of course until at least several decades later, if indeed it ever has. Western-trained physicians possessed the type of expertise linked first to the presence of foreign missionaries in the late nineteenth century; more recently, with the governing power of the colonizer, they have imparted a conflicting set of associations to the popular image of medicine.[20]

One of the most common narratives attesting to the cultural power of medicine in the Korean context concerns the arrival of Protestant missionaries in the late nineteenth century and, specifically, the tale of a successful cure provided to a member of the royal family, with this rhetorical closure leading to the formation of a long-term, productive relationship.[21] This famous story, while central to the foundational myths of Severance Hospital and Yonsei University, now two major institutions of higher education in South Korea, cannot possibly accommodate the conflicting images associated with biomedicine at the close of the war. Beginning with the repatriation process in the fall of 1945, this chapter surveys the diverse approaches adopted with respect to the bodies of returning Koreans for purposes of quarantine, following this series of developments to the cholera outbreaks of spring and summer of 1946 (from May through August), during which the anticipated problem of epidemic disease soon became a reality.[22] In the previous chapter, we surveyed the follow-up activity to this period, during which American authorities recognized the value of relying on TKM practitioners as a contingency measure.

With this strategy, USAMGIK would adopt a deeply ambivalent attitude toward these practitioners, conducting a baseline survey of their numbers (March 1947) and even going so far as to issue licenses to allow them to continue their practice on a limited basis.[23] This approach would also bear a likeness to that undertaken earlier in the century by Japanese authorities, who had sought to reduce the number of practitioners through a series of licensing procedures.[24] For its part, USAMGIK recognized the value of TKM at a time of perceived crisis, assigning practitioners to their village areas as a temporary measure while simultaneously attempting to deal with the problem of disease outbreak (especially enteric disease—typhus, cholera) mainly through quarantine restrictions. At the same time, the production of larger numbers of trained (Korean) doctors and nurses became a high priority, with a partial solution arriving when institutions of higher education began to reopen in August 1946. Here, too, unexpected problems appeared, as class antagonisms buried in the recent past reemerged. Medical students at the newly constituted Seoul National University consisted of members from at least two distinct groups, those resuming their education from Keijo Imperial University (from 1926 to 1945) during the war years and those from neighboring institutions, such as Keijo Medical College.[25]

Ultimately, the conflicts between these distinct populations of medical students, with much of the activity involving medical buildings on the Taehan-no campus, resulted in a temporary shutdown of the "new" university, first in December 1946 and then again in February 1947.[26] This was not simply a conflict over issues of medical pedagogy, and the complex politics of the American occupation—with student representatives from across the political spectrum seeking a voice for their diverse agendas—played a major role. I aim to place these seemingly disparate activities within the framework of a developing pattern, one that witnessed the emergence of biomedicine as a major priority and that was reaffirmed with the outbreak of the Korean War in June 1950. In brief, the response to an outbreak of disease such as cholera in 1946, along with the decision to favor particular types of medical practitioners (promoting biomedicine while licensing and restricting the traditional), both in the field and in the classroom, reflects a series of choices that contributed toward reshaping the priorities of the region to become "South Korea" by August 1948.

In making this claim, I recognize that a significant part of this story involves continuities with the legacy of Japanese colonial medical practice, along with the impact of missionary education. Moreover, the process of division, slow and torturous, cannot neglect the North Korean story, the adjoining region that has had to address many of these same issues and concerns in the act of defining itself. For the latter issue, although I restrict my focus to the South Korean story of an emerging medical community after 1945, I refer readers to the growing scholarship on the North's medical system to indicate comparative developments or points of departure.[27] As for Japan, there is a considerable body of scholarship concerning the use of biomedical science as a formative part of the colonizing process (from 1910 through 1945); more recently, a number of new dissertations and publications have begun to take this work in the direction of gender and reproductive politics, looking at the policing of Korean women and their bodies.[28] Here I will be concerned primarily with the legacy of Japanese models of medical pedagogy and public health, which continued to have an enormous impact on South Korean medical education and public health through at least the late 1960s, a theme that we will encounter frequently.[29]

The transition marking a move from Japanese models to some approximation of American and related international medical practice should not be taken as an abrupt rupture, in other words, but rather as a slow and deliberately paced series of negotiations taking place over at least two to three decades, if not an even longer period of time. The key during the occupation is to recognize the diverse resources initially available with respect to one's body and the treatment of disease, with these options beginning to see a reduction in number following the selection of new choices. South Korean medicine would be shaped significantly by its origins amid this crisis. For medical practitioners, whether Western-trained or TKM, there were new opportunities, with the choices made carrying long-term implications for professional growth or marginalization, although which path lay ahead was by no means certain.

Tracking the Elusive "Harbingers": Mapping Disease Groups (late 1945–August 1946)

The process of repatriation instituted at the major port cities assumed that Koreans wanted to return "home," and it made this same assumption for other subject peoples caught within the disruptive forces of Japanese empire.[30] Even if such a scheme could be worked out, determining an appropriate place of origin for thousands scattered across Northeast and Southeast Asia, this project failed to take into account individual desires, with many hoping to stay in their new locations or to at least have some say in the matter. In the case of many ethnic Koreans to be repatriated from Japan, this question centered on the critical issue of economic survival, as the joint occupations of Japan and Korea greatly restricted their ability to earn a livelihood. Those slated for repatriation were restricted to carrying a bare minimum of goods, forced to leave behind much of what they had acquired while living abroad.[31] Moreover, they returned to a Korean peninsula engulfed in chaos, a place with possibly even less economic activity than occupied Japan, itself in very poor shape at war's end.

Stated in simple terms, the repatriation scheme virtually ensured that there would be resistance from the start, not simply due to the invasive nature of the process but also motivated by economic necessity. If the orderly procession of individuals being counted and ticked off as they entered the port city of Pusan continues to represent a part of our story, such a narrative captures only the official version concerned with inspection, neglecting the vast amounts of undocumented movement that took place simultaneously. On this point, scholars have been calling for a reframing of the existing story of the occupation of Japan for some time, an ambitious project that recognizes the need to look at Korea, Japan, and other occupied territories as a whole.[32] For our story here, the main point of interest lies in the patterns of movement created by the need for basic subsistence, with many Koreans continuing to move between the islands of southern Japan and the Korean peninsula by boat, even after they had been officially accounted for and documented as part of the repatriation process. Koreans were not alone in conducting this sort of activity, but they would receive the brunt of attention in the Japanese context, blamed for a marked increase in black market activity.

If we can momentarily set aside the economic implications of the occupation and a failure to police the movements of certain populations, our focus here rests on how Koreans chose to define themselves by responding to the emergence of a disease crisis in the following year, 1946. Spread typically by the ingestion of contaminated sources of food or water, cholera (*hoyŏlcha*, or *k'ollera*) is a disease associated with a breakdown of civil order and a lack of basic infrastructure, and it tends to appear in the aftermath of human and natural disaster, when clean water and sanitation are stretched to the point of breaking. In this case, the main problem that would appear in 1946 had primarily to do with a cholera outbreak, although typhus would also be heard from in Japan, as the paths of hungry refugees, large numbers of returning military personnel, and the arriving Americans all came to intersect on the peninsula. From the standpoint of perception, too, a problem of equal significance appeared when these issues of disease came to be attributed to the "unclean" bodies of Koreans, especially within the postwar media in Japan and, in many cases, within American military circles.

Reevaluating the Efficacy of American Reforms?

As for the material circumstances leading to a cholera outbreak for much of the following year, 1946 (May–September), the chaotic conditions of the joint occupation contributed to a range of factors, primary among them being a rapid breakdown of infrastructure in the south (food and water supply, sanitation). Dr. Crawford Sams (1902–1994), the American army surgeon responsible for Public Health and Welfare on the Japan/GHQ side (from 1945 to 1951, in Tokyo), acknowledged this possibility from the start, with American troops ordered to permit free passage across the 38th parallel to any persons moving from north to south. According to Sams's account, Russian troops stationed in the border area did not always permit passage out of the northern zone, but the number of individuals either allowed to make this passage or simply doing so via unguarded sections of the border was sufficient to begin placing a strain on the limited resources of the southern zone. We have already seen the system set up at Pusan for the processing of these pools of individuals, and Sams places their point of origin as far north as Manchuria, thereby increasing the possibility for the spread of disease.

But Sams was not concerned with the Korean peninsula but rather with Japan; specifically, his mandate was one of maintaining the health of military personnel in that occupied nation, along with reforming the existing system of medical education. His interest in Koreans lay in their potential as carriers of disease, specifically typhus, as they relocated from their sites of wartime employment. The rough equivalent of the Japanese soldier marching south to Pusan from Manchuria was a Korean laborer, typically a coal miner, headed back to Korea on a boat from the tip of southern Japan, departing from the area near Shimonoseki (southern Honshu). In an oral history interview given at Washington University (St. Louis) in the late 1970s, Sams would single out this group of Koreans as posing the greatest threat to his scheme, noting that this category of refugee did not have the opportunity to maintain cleanliness: "They were all lousy because [in] that kind of situation people can't take baths; they had only the clothes on their backs and so."[33] This retrospective characterization was made not in a spirit of disparagement but one of reaffirming a dominant understanding.

More recently, a newer literature has begun to challenge the claims made by Sams and, more broadly, on behalf of GHQ, in terms of its alleged accomplishments in fields such as public health. There has been a tendency, particularly in the case of the GHQ occupation, to assign too much credit to biomedicine, adopting a critical position toward the entire spectrum of prewar and wartime Japanese civil institutions. This approach had sought to make space for a celebration of American-backed reforms, replacing local practice with the new during the course of the occupation. In "Typhus in Occupied Japan, 1945–46: an Epidemiological Study," Chris Aldous does not fault the introduction of American practice but instead makes an argument for a much higher degree of continuity, suggesting that any success came only through reliance on existing forms of public health practice.[34] In the Korean context, this line of argument fits as well, especially as the USAMGIK obsession with maintaining quarantine in the port areas holds numerous echoes with Japanese practice during the preceding period. We also know that Japanese health experts such as Shiga Kiyoshi were consulted, drawing on their expertise from the preceding colonial period.

Before we return to the USAMGIK, it is worth recalling once more the antagonisms generated by movements of these groups of Korean refugees, especially those illegally reentering Japan after being repatriated. In "Invisible Immigrants," Tessa Morris-Suzuki enumerates the reasons Koreans felt compelled to return, including the purchase of goods and resources scarce in Korea, as well as to satisfy basic economic needs.[35] As she points out further, a number of these ethnic Koreans were born in and had lived in Japan for their entire lives and did not necessarily identify with Korea or regard it as their home. From a strictly economic standpoint, the circumstances of the repatriation were extremely harsh, permitting those departing to bring with them only 1,000 yen, this being roughly equivalent to the purchase price of a half bushel of rice.[36] Under these conditions, Morris-Suzuki claims that many families adopted a strategy of selecting one member to repatriate first, with that individual planning to return in the event that he or she found conditions in Korea unsuitable in the course of setting up a household.

This category of "harbingers," as Morris-Suzuki labels them, were regarded as the ones primarily responsible for creating problems for the occupation authorities on the GHQ side. Not only typhus but also cholera was attributed to the patterns of movement of Koreans and Taiwanese primarily to, but also from, Japan. For his part, Dr. Sams was quite comfortable with this characterization, especially for the cholera outbreak in Korea, remarking that "two cases of cholera unfortunately got ashore at Pusan from a group returning by ship from China," dating his remark to approximately late 1945.[37] He goes on to detail the spread of the disease in a pattern approximating the major rail lines between Seoul and Pusan, a claim we shall examine shortly.[38] To be clear, though, our interest lies not in the ethnic and nationalist tensions between Japan and its former imperial subjects or even in establishing a firm basis for evaluating the reliability of Sams's account. What we need to emphasize instead is the use of the perceived cholera crisis as justification for a series of medical reforms to follow—infrastructural (promoting biomedicine through vaccination campaigns and DDT dusting) and statistical (promoting the collection of vital statistics and demography)—during the remainder of the occupation, along with its likely impact on the formation of a South Korean medical community after 1948.

In contrast to Sams, Willard does not even mention the cholera outbreak in his retrospective account, focusing instead on material issues of infrastructure and the possibility of typhus. From his perspective, the major issue was the simple possibility of an epidemic, with the specific disease itself representing a lesser concern: "Typhus was feared as the major problem during the winter [of 1945 to 1946]," with smallpox and malaria also receiving a great deal of attention in advance.[39] Given this outlook, his approach lay with acquiring and distributing the necessary implements in bulk, the "DDT, dust guns, power dusters, vaccine, syringes, and needles" to mount a vigorous and effective campaign.[40] For hospitals and clinics, similarly, the needs were just as basic, with a marked lack of the goods required for even normal maintenance: "coal, food, drugs, dressings, paint, window glass, soap, instruments."[41] Closer to the scene than his Tokyo colleague, Willard recognized that he could not anticipate every scenario, and his confidence lay in a different direction, establishing the organization and supply lines that could convey materials to the site when called on.

Cholera and the Biopolitics of Crisis (April 1946–September 1946): Mobilizing Reforms in the South

Making its presence felt in increments, news of a cholera outbreak began to surface in the weekly and monthly bulletins issued by USAMGIK in mid-May of 1946, with the overall pattern of incidents suggesting an outbreak situated in or near the port city of Pusan.[42] Tracking reports from this possible source, the bulletins tend to suggest a pattern of movement northwest across the peninsula, possibly following the movements of refugees in this direction. A particular problem at this point was the issue of the dealing with the temporary border, the 38th parallel, as disease does not respect the human markers that hold enormous significance in political affairs. Most likely, cholera affected the northern zone at this time, with many of the border provinces of the south severely affected and with the outbreak peaking at some point in July 1946, gradually diminishing to reach its end by approximately September.[43]

The cross-border issue is difficult to track precisely because of a lack of reliable reports, but certainly those dealing with the disease in the southern zone believed that their northern counterparts were similarly afflicted. The two patrons, the Americans and the Soviets, also became involved in the issue when the United States sought to purchase a supply of chlorine for water purification, with the majority of facilities for chlorine production located in the northern zone.[44] The Soviets agreed to the exchange only when the Americans pointed out that they maintained a similar hold over the rice supply and might easily cut off the northern zone if the request for chlorine were not granted in a gesture of reciprocity.[45] If this incident underscores the delicate relationship between the two zones, emphasizing their interdependence previously as a nation and then as a colonial space constructed for Japanese purposes, the division of the two zones further exacerbated this kind of problem.

In putting together the elements of a cholera control program (*k'ollera ŏkche p'ŭrogŭraem*), occupation authorities had to be aware of these systemic issues, meeting subsistence needs in two critical areas—supplies of clean water and food to reduce the spread—while figuring out how to minimize the impact of the disease.

Concerning these two issues, food and water, environmental factors intervened and made the cholera problem even more difficult to contain. A lack of chemical fertilizer, which had previously been supplied by the northern-based chemical industry, resulted in a reduced grain supply in 1946, with the harvest for the year coming later than usual.[46] In turn, the rainy season (*changma*) brought with it heavier than usual rains in June 1946, flooding many rice paddies and overwhelming the irrigation system designed to channel water to the rice paddies. The rains serve to explain in part delays to the harvest, as well as contributing to the reduction in agricultural yield at the back end. Whether the loss of chemical fertilizer placed a greater emphasis on the use of alternative sources, such as "night soil," is not known, but the cholera outbreak almost certainly coincided with the arrival of the rains, making this reasonable ground for speculation. In brief, the warm, wet months of June and July, with food stocks dwindling, refugees on the move, and sources of clean water very scarce, saw some of the highest numbers registered for those affected by disease.[47]

In quantitative terms, the problem of material lack gave occupation authorities sufficient justification to begin pursuing a program of reforms with long-term implications. Moreover, the lack of grain and sources of potable water provided grounds for a critique of the Japanese colonial infrastructure, seeking to distinguish the American presence ideologically and materially from the work of its predecessor. In the case of water, for example, the Japanese had devoted a good deal of attention to locating sources for artesian wells as well as providing updated forms of sanitation to urban locations. Indeed, this type of work fit quite well within the overall scheme characterized by Gi-Wook Shin and Michael Robinson as "colonial modernity," that is, constructing a refurbished colonial reality from those elements designed to foster an ethic of indebtedness.[48] Rather than limit resources available to colonial subjects, such an approach produced a new kind of colony, one fostering an ideal of eager industrial workers with its economic growth based on ambitious technological schemes.

With the arrival of Americans, this technological set of ideals came to an abrupt end; with respect to medical practice, the occupation authority began to enforce the distinction almost immediately with Ordinance #1, which abolished the Japanese system of attaching its medical services to the police bureau.[49] Famously, this style of practice had only added to the negative associations of medicine and quarantine, meaning that it was the colonial police who had been largely responsible for monitoring any signs of disease.[50] The establishment of a "new" Bureau of Public Health and Welfare took place beginning in September 1945, with the name officially changing as of late October 1945.[51] More than a mere change of labels, the new agency took shape under the authority of Ordinance #18 (October 27, 1945), and the language of the proclamation mobilized the notion of reaching out at times of emergency and crisis, aiding those parties requiring assistance. Again, this is not to say that the occupation was necessarily qualitatively different from its Japanese predecessor in its practice, but at least it was highly conscious of crafting its distinct image.

In theory, the Bureau was well prepared to anticipate many of the problems that soon appeared, but a lack of resources and trained personnel resulted in shortages and the need for individual actors to take on multiple roles.[52] An early attempt at establishing a baseline nutritional survey, for example, was canceled prematurely for this very reason, losing a potential source of data that might have been valuable the following year when cholera would become a major problem.[53] The dissolution of the police bureau also resulted in a great deal of confusion as different bureaucratic organizations were no longer clear about their individual responsibilities. Previously, everything from prostitution to public health enforcement had fallen under a single umbrella, and now many of these areas had to be dealt with separately, handed out to distinct bodies. In the short term, the result was a significant time lag built into any scheme of enforcement, with a strong tendency to rely on the status quo.

When reports of a disease outbreak first begin to trickle in—variously reported as dating to roughly April or May of 1946—there was then a significant delay before the introduction of any systematic approach to the problem.[54] In keeping with the Sams account, the greatest concentration of cholera cases appeared in the southeast, suggesting Pusan as a possible point of origin, although this was by no means the only area affected. For the duration of the outbreak, the two neighboring provinces comprising the southeast, Kyŏngsang-bukto and Kyŏngsang-namdo (north and south Kyŏngsang) were among the hardest hit, receiving a corresponding degree of attention from occupation authorities. The official account from the perspective of American military medicine suggests a relationship to a corresponding outbreak taking place in China at about the same time, with Korean refugees bringing the disease along with them. Despite the precautions introduced in the form of quarantine, cholera made its way up the peninsula.

The delays in introducing whole-scale measures likely had more to do with the problem of resource scarcity than with any indecision on the part of the incoming medical authority. The previous year the American military had taken control over production facilities left behind by the Japanese, meaning that the Bureau had access to at least a limited supply of vaccine. However, the issue of finding personnel with sufficient training to operate the available facilities limited the reliance on these sources, and a good deal of vaccine had to be imported from nearby Japan, underscoring a pattern that we will see again later. Before turning to the question of how the distribution of new medicines was received by the population, it is important to recognize that any intervention was both familiar and disruptive. To begin with, the establishment of control over the medical supply had brought with it new restrictions concerning the right of Korean practitioners to sell their own remedies (Ordinance #62, March 1946). Moreover, the formal control of medicines under the bureau was declared only as of May 1946, roughly simultaneous to the outbreak, suggesting that control over these valuable resources was tenuous at best.

The decision to institute a regionwide vaccination program in June 1946, while well motivated, represented a response to an acute situation that was nearly impossible to execute in practice. Occupation authorities had just begun to assert control over a limited number of production facilities, including the National Vaccine Laboratory, with a corresponding lack of staff to replace Japanese personnel who had recently departed.[55] With the outbreak reaching its highest numbers in July, USAMGIK opted to begin importing its sources for the cholera vaccine, with much of this material deriving from Japan, although sources also point to supplies arriving from the United States.[56] Even assuming that there was a sufficient quantity of doses to treat the population, this development raised the next question, the logistical problem of how to administer the vaccine to a large number of individuals quickly and effectively. At least officially, the occupation claimed success in performing this act, reaching a significant majority of those living south of the 38th parallel.

On the ground, the story was quite different, and more recent accounts have begun to acknowledge this reality, with at least one scholar characterizing the public health regime as "at best, a holding operation" for the duration of the occupation.[57] Rather than vaccination, the key practice for much of June and July was a comprehensive effort to restrict movement of all kinds, not only placing physical barriers in the form of quarantine at points of entry but even seeking to limit refugees' ability to travel by rail or on foot. In principle, this policy initiative made perfect sense, but, again, it led to immense practical difficulties as the repatriation process was ongoing and a second flow of refugees from north to south was taking place. Moreover, the perceived sources of the spread of the disease, contaminated food and water, tended to be associated with large clusters of individuals, often taking the form of public gatherings. In the context of the time, this meant that USAMGIK might even seek limitations on activities requiring group assembly or on religious ceremonies, such as marriages or funeral gatherings.[58] In short, the travel restrictions carried with them political overtones of limiting movement and expression, something that gave pause to occupation authorities.

Late in the previous year, USAMGIK had announced in conjunction with the Soviets that the occupation would continue for a defined period of time in the form of a trusteeship, with a decision to be postponed until the parties could agree what to do about Korea.[59] The news, officially labeled the "Moscow Agreement," called for a five-year period of joint custody and led to numerous antitrusteeship demonstrations in the southern zone. While USAMGIK maintained its authority, it became increasingly aware of its perceived role as an oppressor, particularly as circumstances worsened in the summer with the cholera outbreak. For example, the reduced grain harvest, in part a by-product of the heavy rains and flooding, required that the Korean National Police step in as a means of collecting grain, offering minimal compensation to farmers. In the estimation of historian Allan Millett, this policy "looked like confiscation" to farmers and fueled suspicions that the Americans were not that different from the Japanese who had preceded them.[60]

Collectively, the public health measures that followed—travel restrictions, mass inoculation for cholera as new supplies of vaccine arrived, and spraying—tended to reinforce the image of a new colonizer, one motivated by vigorous forms of hygiene policing and enforcement. Despite the increased vigilance, however, the disease continued to make its way northward, and travelers continued to evade the inspection of the bureau. In total, an estimated 15,000 Koreans were infected, leading to deaths in the range of about 10,000 to 11,000 individuals by September 1946, before the outbreak finally began to wane. The change in season, with the arrival of cooler weather, certainly helped to alleviate the situation, as did reduced numbers of potential bodies to infect: The epidemic effectively burned itself out, having reached its peak in the late summer. Along with political turmoil, USAMGIK had a number of related problems to address and recognized the need to take its public health considerations much more seriously in the future.

In reexamining the disease crisis, it is critical to recognize the significance of framing. The cholera outbreak of summer 1946 was accorded the status of a crisis precisely because it restricted the American military in its operations, and this holds true especially for the potential to disrupt the functioning of the larger, regional occupation (GHQ). This is not to say that cholera did not kill individuals, but the disease was one familiar to many Koreans and did not necessarily inspire the same fear there that it did in American military circles. In turn, the myopic perceptions of American actors did not mean that they were unwilling to respond to their Korean counterparts, however, and their well-intentioned actions sometimes led to positive achievements. In particular, if there was a problem with disease, this translated as an acute need for greater numbers of trained Korean doctors and nurses, a problem to be addressed by providing greater access to higher education. This was an issue that was addressed by opening up schools as early as March 1946, a development covered extensively in Michael Seth's *Education Fever* and by reopening and increasing access to higher education as of August 1946.

The "Crisis" in Retrospect: The Elision of Historical Precedents?

Rather than establish the circumstances of the terminal point of the cholera outbreak in late 1946, our concern here should focus on the issue of what impact the selection of an interpretive frame had on subsequent policy. The Korean peninsula has a lengthy history of dealing with epidemic disease, one easily traced through Korean and Chinese texts; indeed, Dr. Shin Dong-Won of KAIST has written an entire volume devoted exclusively to cholera.[61] Working from a short-term trajectory (late 1930s to 1945) quite distinct from that of its local counterparts, USAMGIK retained little, if any, historical consciousness when dealing with issues of disease and scarce resources, tending to read these concerns through the immediate precedent of Japanese public health, which it regarded an abject failure.[62] With the waning of the 1946 crisis, the military authority was eager to claim a measure of "success" for its own efforts, and our pursuit shifts to one of following the trend toward even greater reliance on Western medicine and, along with this, the confidence associated with the ability to mobilize interventions on a mass scale.

The framing of the occupation as an external or regional effort, as opposed to the Korean peninsula in isolation, therefore becomes critical to understanding the American military mind-set, preoccupied as it was with limiting the spread of disease by any means. The problem of "harbingers" pops up frequently in the literature concerning the GHQ occupation and, with this recognition, the realization that the crisis was never simply a matter for Koreans alone but, rather, a much wider regional affair affecting much of Northeast Asia. Moreover, the concern affected American policy in China and Taiwan as well, although to expand the discussion to include this material would require a much lengthier look at possible routes of migration.[63] For now, suffice it to say that contemporary accounts of disease issues generally focused on the power and effectiveness of large-scale infrastructural interventions, attesting to the ability to reduce the numbers of individuals affected.[64] Although these developments reflect an American viewpoint, it is not difficult to speculate about their possible impact on Korean actors with the transition in government to come shortly, beginning in August 1948.

Precedents Established by a Crisis Scenario

In other words, the pattern of interventions introduced under American military authority helped to establish the type of precedent that might soon be adopted by an independent ROK. This is not an argument for strict causation by any means and is instead a claim for a high degree of path dependency introduced under the conditions of a crisis. Dr. Willard, nominally in charge of these unusual circumstances, acknowledged the many problems caused by his lack of familiarity with the context, even when operating with good intentions. The decision to remove the presence of the colonial police from health matters was covered under the very first ordinance issued by the military government (October 1945), for example, based on the "conviction . . . that public health is not a police function."[65] Even as this gesture met with considerable approval from Korean doctors, Willard soon recognized that it seriously disrupted his ability to collect information and to keep track of the presence of communicable disease. The figure of the village police officer, if enormously controversial, had nonetheless served as "the sanitary inspector and [had] supplied health intelligence," along with the regular duties.[66]

Aware of Korean sensitivities, Willard appears cautious here not to praise the Japanese system, recognizing the enormous discomfort created by a health regime enforced "under police domination and by police methods."[67] At the same time, he laments the loss of the information supplied by these ground-based actors, who had reported to lower levels of government, essential in any outbreak of disease. In the short term, Willard characterizes the response to the ordinance as one of a communications breakdown, with police distancing themselves from public health activities as requested by the ordnance. From his perspective, though, the act of compliance led to an even more significant problem, at least potentially: a major disruption to the public health network, "particularly in rural areas, long before any substitute organization could be created."[68]

This recurring pattern of explicit rejection of Japanese models, while remarking on the utility of their design, characterizes many of Willard's remarks from the period, underscoring his ambivalence. Other American actors, as we will see shortly, would make observations with a comparable focus when approaching the issue of population, rejecting the more conspicuous and crude interventions mobilized by Japanese police and health officials, while seeking to preserve the underlying functions motivating such actions. In fact, many of the criticisms of the occupation's health policies have focused on precisely this point, the continuity with Japanese precedents. But the issue is not as simple as a whole-scale rejection of one set of practices in favor of another, as the 1947 survey of TKM practitioners indicates. Still, the acute need for materials, along with greater numbers of trained personnel, meant that USAMGIK had to regulate not only personnel but also the market for drugs, whether traditional or pharmaceutical, curtailing the ability to prepare and sell traditional remedies in an outdoor setting.

Together, these two major issues (personnel and materials) went a long way toward granting greater power to biomedicine, as USAMGIK first sought to reopen schools at all levels (March 1946), with this gesture including medical schools at the university level (August 1946). Although this gesture would prove popular in the long run, it raised concerns about establishing Korean control and specifically concerns about which groups of local actors would gain access to and subsequent control over the institutions. Next, with drugs and materials in short supply, the temporary solution lay in a series of improvised moves, including seizing and deploying stocks left behind by Japan, along with establishing new supply lines through American bases situated nearby in the region. Dr. Willard characterized this frenzied activity as "scrounging," performing a series of bureaucratic tasks when the time might be better spent on "directing the manufacture of biological products or in training Koreans to do laboratory work."[69] "Scrounging" would thus connote an entire range of activities; specifically, this could also mean an officer gathering "material from other Army units to rehabilitate laboratory equipment, or to make culture media, in waiting for a jeep to take him to the laboratory, in making out payrolls for his Korean employees."[70]

In Willard's narrative, this type of activity occupies a disproportionate amount of the time devoted to health, suggesting that bureaucratic routine was far more common than actual encounters with patients or performing related tasks: "The time required for administrative work far overshadowed that devoted to medical work."[71] Similarly, although he refers frequently to local personnel in the context of handing over basic tasks or functions—"Koreans were found and trained to take over operating responsibilities as quickly as possible"—his account lacks any real sense of these personnel as individuals, characterizing them only in collective terms.[72] Given Willard's role, this type of descriptive convention is understandable, in that he was occupied with the task of bureaucratic oversight; but, unfortunately, the attitude typified a good deal of USAMGIK's dealings with its counterparts.

Moreover, it suggests that the formation of a subsequent South Korean public health was very much shaped by these circumstances of crisis and material lack. The majority of the trained Korean personnel (nurses, doctors, *chogyo*) at this time would have prior experience of Japanese training, with the obvious exception of those passing through Severance Union Hospital. The transition to newer models of medicine came incrementally, and, despite its public rejection of its predecessor, USAMGIK replicated many of the choices made under colonialism. Along with this pattern of continuity comes a second issue, the question of an origin point for a "South Korean" public health, given the formal declaration of independence in August 1948. The type of large-scale interventions associated with a public health crisis, to be followed shortly by the circumstances of the Korean War, reminds us that the ROK military served as one of the major providers of health care at a time when such an entity barely existed at the state level. Willard's reports cite the opportunity for limited numbers of these Koreans to begin traveling abroad for study, and the experience of war would soon provide rapid exposure in the form of clinical experience.

This account does not necessarily contradict a historiography that celebrates the accomplishments of Korean medicine over the long term (from 1876 through the present), one seeking to establish a pattern of continuity, linking the late-nineteenth-century appearance of Western biomedicine on the peninsula with the events of the late 1940s. It does, however, recognize such a narrative as a construction celebrating the accomplishments of the nation and, as such, one calling for interrogation. Limited numbers of trained medical personal and medical supplies created the conditions that first produced a tentative, bureaucratic structure resembling a South Korean public health, and these origins lead to a very different kind of story. In the aftermath of epidemic outbreak, moreover, the concerns of dealing with a growing population began to create a need for the resumption of demographic activity, another area that had been dominated by the Japanese.[73] With much of the population based in rural areas, this proved a formidable challenge.

Mobilizing Demography and Social Science (September 1948–)

With a lengthy history of written records on the peninsula, the accumulated data for tracking population was substantial, covering the colonial period, along with much of the preceding Chosŏn period. The emergence of demographic concerns was not an entirely new issue, therefore, although it was mobilized as "new" by visiting social scientists who sought to implement reforms to the methods employed. These issues were a frequent topic of discussion during the late colonial period, with Japanese efforts aimed at limiting population growth, a development detailed by Dr. Sonja Kim of Binghamton University in her recent dissertation, "Limiting Birth."[74] Moreover, the series of internal migrations associated with the postwar further increased the pressure to have measures in place to be able to take a reliable estimate of the population, a useful index in any set of circumstances but especially at a time linked with the formation of a new nation.

The benefits of undertaking such a project were numerous, given the activities associated with national renewal, including the establishment of the armed forces, the need to assess the population for taxation purposes, and any number of related bureaucratic functions. Moreover, the problems of public health and disease dating to the occupation period underscored the need for knowledge about the movements of individuals, not simply for the purposes of record keeping but also as a measure of public health. Although Japanese records for these purposes were extensive, they soon came under attack, both from USAMGIK and from the visiting fellows of the Rockefeller Foundation, who argued that they represented only a partial, incomplete data set. In particular, the *koseki*, or household registry, became the focus of intense scrutiny, with its critics arguing that the registry, kept at the family or ancestral home, failed in a fundamental way: It linked the individual to the residence, without tracking his or her subsequent actions, a fatal flaw in a site where the 1930s and 1940s had brought massive migration.

The Rockefeller Report (March 1950)

The motivation underlying these matters was not simply one of a state interested in the whereabouts of its citizens but rather a new postcolonial state hoping to keep the incidence of disease outbreak to a minimum. The recent cholera, smallpox, and typhus outbreaks of the occupation were still very much in the minds of Koreans as they began to establish their own public health institutions. With this in mind, a Rockefeller–sponsored visit in the fall of 1948 (September to December), including several prominent demography experts, established contact with the latest forms of American social science. This was not a visit made exclusively to South Korea; it included the entire span of what was still characterized as the "Far East"—including Japan, Taiwan, Korea, the Republic of China, Indonesia, and the Philippines—reflecting American interests in assessing prospects for friendly relations and economic development. Along with public health, the visitors, with Princeton University's OPR (Office of Population Research) researchers Frank Notestein and Irene Taeuber among them, looked carefully at the demographic factors contributing to population growth, which would become a concern over the next two decades.

In keeping with the private rhetoric of the occupation, the Rockefeller team members appeared largely comfortable with the legacy of the Japanese public health system, arguing that it had dramatically reduced mortality, effectively holding major outbreaks of disease in check. These comments were directed specifically at a reduction in the infant mortality rate, with a follow-up offering qualified praise, noting that a "consequence of a reasonably sound and efficient economic and political exploitation was a decline in the general level of mortality."[75] "Japanese efficiency," for example, had managed to limit disease of epidemic proportions to a great extent, although many conditions "remained endemic." The concern with mortality was directed less at public health issues than at assessing the overall rate of population increase, which had continued on its upward slope, making it a "classic example of the demographic tragedy of colonial rule."[76]

This last remark can be explained in terms of the conflict between a growing population and the inadequate employment opportunities made available to Koreans during the mid-1930s. With an estimated 80 percent of the population working in the agricultural sector, much of it based in the south, there were few opportunities for class mobility. Even finding subsistence-level employment, whether in agriculture or in one of the larger cities, meant a lengthy search, with many Koreans forced to migrate abroad in search of work. Written in late 1949, this characterization captures again the difficult circumstances described at the beginning of this chapter, with Koreans forced to repatriate regardless of poor economic conditions. From this perspective, migration for the purpose of obtaining industrial jobs in Japan was much less about "push" than "pull," with survival furnishing the necessary incentive. Moreover, the Rockefeller team members could see no short-term solution to the issue of population increase on the peninsula, as "no Western means of family limitation is appropriate to the living conditions and the cultural levels in the Korean villages," and prospects for domestic economic development looked poor.[77]

Family planning would become a central part of the ROK state's strategy within less than two decades (by 1964), but it would require the energy and enthusiasm of a domestic community of Korean scholars to mobilize the necessary resources. In addition, Rockefeller staff members would not have known that a portion of the Korean population had already been exposed to these new ideas, including a select group of women based in urban Seoul. The latest work of Japanese sexologists would have reached the colonies during the late colonial period in the 1930s, although it is difficult to determine how many adopted the recommended forms of practice. In her work *Colonizing Sex* (2003), Sabine Fruhstuck includes the example of the Ota ring, one of the first IUD (intrauterine device) technologies, remarking that it would reach the cities of Taipei and Seoul, although she acknowledges that the extent of its penetration into the market lies beyond her focus.[78] At this early point, the Rockefeller concerns aired here have to be viewed primarily in terms of the occupation of Japan and the overall effort to restore a peacetime level of subsistence to Northeast Asia.

It is also worth mentioning a further limitation of the Rockefeller survey: its lack of penetration into village life. With a brief duration (September to December 1948), the survey visits covered a wide area and acknowledged from the outset a desire to take a broad approach that would necessarily miss a great deal of country-specific details. If it is not surprising that Rockefeller missed traces of a new population concern among elites in passing through South Korea, it is startling that it largely omitted mention of its counterpart, abortion and other "traditional" methods of population control. The category of "spontaneous abortion," along with a range of herbal methods, would represent the target of a great deal of effort on the part of ROK family planning workers within about two decades, and it is unlikely that this culture emerged only in the aftermath of the Korean War. A more likely scenario is that the Rockefeller visitors could spend only limited time among rural populations and could not be expected to notice every aspect of daily living, even something as critical as this practice.

Even with omissions like this, the Rockefeller Report remains fascinating for an on-the-ground look at South Korea material conditions immediately following independence and just prior to the outbreak of the Korean War (September 1948 through early June 1950). If the document remains at a distance from the new ROK government, it still serves as a useful framework through which to discuss many of the concerns that would emerge after the war, especially in terms of mobilizing new forms of social science. The nation described here remains rural, celebrating the "idealization of the life of the peasant," even as the report anticipates a different future.[79] Careful in its critique, the report also praises the efforts of the new government, along with the USAMGIK, arguing that the combined efforts of the two bodies had continued the positive trend of reducing mortality, even if this has resulted in a population problem. At least implicitly, some of the blame is attributed to the ROK government, for it favored these demographic trends, believing that much of its power lay in growing numbers, a development that Rockefeller hoped to reverse.

At the time, a South Korean public health system, as limited in scope as it might have been, appeared highly similar to what had been in place roughly three years earlier. The number of doctors was extremely low—outnumbered by TKM practitioners in some locations—although the reopening of medical schools was already helping to improve the situation. Still, the majority of graduates were Koreans with substantial Japanese training, and Japanese medical models continued to inform clinical practice. Contact and encounter with the state's medical system was largely confined to a few urban areas, with the majority of doctors residing in these areas. In a practical sense, the burden of preventive care often fell on traditional practitioners, who remained the favored choice of many. Of these developments, the critical one was not the similarity of the circumstances but the move toward independence, meaning that Koreans could now self-determine with respect to their medical and health options.

With independence would come further debates about the logistics of a national approach to medicine, if not any substantive material change on issues like access and health insurance, concerns that would be addressed only much later. Along with the major disease concerns—including here chronic or endemic conditions such as leprosy, tuberculosis, and the enteric outbreaks detailed here—the issue of identity remained on the table, although the public character of this issue frequently varied in its intensity. Traditional medicine continued on the path toward a marginal status in this period, even while figuring prominently in the self-concept of the broader medical community. Biomedicine, on the other hand, especially as practiced by its Korean practitioners, had to address the problem of its origins, deriving from Western missionary resources, as well as the more obvious and prickly precedent of Japanese colonialism. If its effects were regarded as positive, it nonetheless remained largely unfamiliar, and it retained a provisional status as something borrowed or imported.

The first of these two issues changed in less than two years, with the arrival of the Korean War, bringing with it widespread destruction and an immediate need for medical relief work of all kinds. The United States brought its mobile medical and surgical teams along with the better-known military intervention and, moreover, was augmented by an international team of medical experts, with the most prominent of these deriving from a set of Scandinavian actors, including Norway, Sweden, and Denmark. At least in the short term, the issue of prior training and status receded as a concern for the Korean doctors and nurses involved, many of whom gained valuable clinical experience working under these challenging conditions. With contingency and material lack serving as the baseline conditions, it became far easier to intervene in the body to do quick repair, leaving other questions for the period of postoperative recovery.

3 "From Minneapolis to Seoul": Transforming Surgery, Clinical Practice, and Professional Identity at Seoul National University Hospital, 1954–1968

Treating Tuberculosis: Limiting the Impact of Chronic Disease (1955)

When Dr. Lee Chan-Bum (1915–1967) began work for his master's degree at a U.S. Army base hospital in Masan in the early 1950s, the focus of his research, the long-term effects of tuberculosis (*kyŏrhaek*), represented one of the greatest threats to public health in South Korea.[1] Dr. Lee, a surgeon affiliated with the Republic of Korea Army (ROKA), was interested in exploring techniques for the removal of lesions on lung tissue, excising damaged areas to permit ease of breathing, and, potentially, to return the patient to a better quality of life. At the time, this style of chest surgery represented the state of the art; moreover, it offered significant comfort to a developing nation recovering from the destructive effects of the Korean War.[2] In fact, tuberculosis posed a threat sufficiently dangerous that when the U.S. Eighth Army contributed financial assistance toward the construction of a new facility to be based on the campus of Yonsei University (1957), the site was devoted exclusively to this type of chest surgery, bearing the label the "Memorial Chest Surgery Hospital."[3]

Dr. Lee, along with his close friend and partner, Dr. Lee Young-Gyun (1921–1994), was among a new generation of South Korean physicians and practitioners who found their careers dramatically transformed by an infusion of postwar funding and material assistance deriving from both American and international sources.[4] Less than five years after completing his master's thesis in 1955, Lee Chan-Bum found himself in America, completing part of a visiting surgical residency at the Veterans Administration (VA) Hospital in Minneapolis, granted the luxury of time to study and learn the latest available techniques in clinical medicine.[5] His placement in Minnesota, moreover, was not accidental, as it coincided with Dr. Lee's previous training as an ROKA military surgeon and was designed to meet the needs of a comprehensive aid project taking place between the University of Minnesota and Seoul National University (SNU) under the sponsorship of the International Cooperation Administration (ICA), the American agency responsible for coordinating technical diplomacy.[6] Covering three broad subject areas—including medicine (nursing, veterinary medicine, and parasitology), agriculture, and engineering—the "Minnesota Project" (1954–1962) radically overhauled clinical practice and pedagogy at the South Korean national university, effectively making it one of the leading facilities for medical education.[7]

Although Dr. Lee's prior experience extended to opening the chest cavity and handling diseased lung tissue, he was soon working with the most invasive and radical surgical techniques of the period, learning a version of the open-heart surgical techniques previously worked out at the University of Minnesota under a surgical team headed by renowned cardiac surgeon Dr. C. Walton Lillehei (1918–1999).[8] In other words, Dr. Lee underwent a rapid personal transformation from performing a series of fairly conventional lung surgeries to recruiting and leading members of his own open heart surgery team in slightly less than a decade.[9] This type of radical career transformation was made possible in part through the careful coordination of the Minnesota Project, which oversaw the individual study tours of South Korean personnel in Minneapolis, as well as the physical rehabilitation of the infrastructure and medical pedagogy at Seoul National University Hospital.[10] By 1968, this facility had assembled its own thoracic surgery unit, a team of skilled physicians and nurses capable of handling a wide range of heart cases.[11]

Transforming Professional and Personal Identity

The use of the label "thoracic surgery" in South Korea context at this early date highlights the ambition and scale of the program envisioned by these Korean actors, who took great pride in overhauling their institution and its practice. At the same time, the label conveniently elides the dense nexus of historical tensions present at the site: Seoul National University Hospital continued to be regarded as essentially a "Japanese" facility by many of the American visitors associated with the Minnesota Project, and this pejorative label appeared as late as the mid-1960s, referring specifically to particular aspects of clinical practice as well as to an autocratic pedagogical style attributed to certain groups of elite Korean doctors.[12] For nearly two decades, the hospital site functioned as the centerpiece of the Japanese imperial university in colonial Korea, Keijo Imperial University (1926–1945), with most entering classes of medical students made up of approximately two-thirds to three-quarters Japanese nationals, individuals training to become doctors to care for a growing settler population.[13] Under the circumstances, the hospital carried with it an uncomfortable legacy in the postliberation period (from 1948 on), even as it would become one of South Korea's leading medical institutions.

In turn, when visiting University of Minnesota faculty members described the hospital as "Japanese," this constructed label carried with it a range of potential meanings, but most specifically with reference to the style of medical practice characterizing South Korean health care. In brief, the hospital bore all the signs of its lengthy colonial past, continuing to employ many of the methods common to the German academic medicine of the late nineteenth century, which the Japanese had passed on to their colonies.[14] It was not common to take tissue samples from patients, for example, nor did the hospital perform autopsies with any consistency.[15] Anatomy lectures typically involved demonstrations with a single human subject on display, but medical students themselves had very little opportunity to engage with the human body until after they had graduated.[16] The doctor typically held an autocratic role, standing beyond question, and this style of presentation frequently carried over to the lecture theater, where the professor served as a source of knowledge but did not routinely entertain questions from students.

Collectively, these American perceptions have to be subjected to careful scrutiny, as they clearly reflect an external construction of the Japanese legacy, roughly a decade following South Korean independence. Nevertheless, this issue of professional identity in transition is a useful one: The hospital site was itself undergoing a rapid transformation, and this process affected not just Seoul National University but also its close neighbor and competitor, Yonsei University, the recent product of a joint relationship formed between Yonhi College and Severance Union Hospital in the second half of the 1950s, providing an additional source of rapid change in South Korean biomedicine.[17] Beginning in 1957, medical students at SNU experienced a new regime of clinical training modeled on that of their international peers, with the introduction of new professional categories—the clerk (1957), the intern (1958), and the resident (1959).[18] At the level of material practice, new equipment and lab facilities at the hospital meant the availability of rapid on-site analysis for tissue samples and blood work, thereby transforming the body of the patient into an object of biomedical research.

From its inception, the Minnesota Project intended to follow precisely along these lines, with the emphasis shifting from an initial focus on Minneapolis (1954–1957) to Seoul (1958–1962) during the second half of the decade. This approach meant that the early period was dominated by a focus on material and infrastructural improvements to the hospital site from 1954 to 1957, while Korean doctors and nurses studied at the Minneapolis campus. Coinciding with their return, the second portion of the program shifted to pedagogy and the implementation of a new clinical regime, with returning students teaching their peers who had not yet had the opportunity to go abroad. Along with thoracic surgery, neurosurgery, under the direction of Dr. Lyle French (1915–2004), was among the specialties to be introduced, and Korean surgeons were performing their own procedures on an independent basis by as early as the start of the new decade, translating their newly acquired skills into surgical practice.[19]

For young doctors like Lee Chan-Bum and Lee Young-Gyun, the transformation in their surgical practice—the ability to go much further than their predecessors in terms of planning and pursuing an independent biomedical research agenda—was by no means a straightforward one, and they were working frequently in the absence of any firm institutional or ethical guidelines as to the treatment of human bodies. Moreover, both men experienced a second, equally important, transition, leaving behind their previous identity as "*Choson-in*," or Japanese colonial subjects, for a new professional identity as elites in an independent South Korea. This was not a simple matter of shedding their skin for a new identity but rather a complicated process of negotiating, practicing, and living simultaneously multiple forms of identity; certainly "Japanese" medical practice continued to inform the South Korean hospital site well into the decade of the 1960s.[20] The lived experience of encountering and embracing this unstable form of identity is frequently missing from similar accounts in which the post–Korean War transition to newer medical models simply takes place in a rapid and unproblematic fashion.[21]

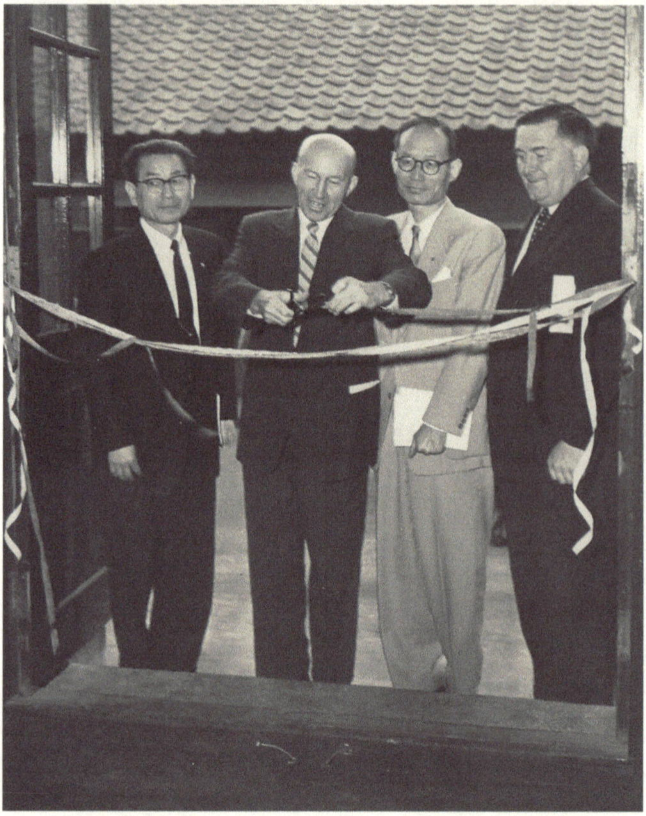

Dr. Arthur Schneider (second from left) of the University of Minnesota at a ribbon-cutting ceremony held in Seoul during the early stages of the Minnesota Project (1954 to 1962). Dr. Schneider had previously worked in South Korea as a forestry specialist with the USAMGIK in the late 1940s during the American occupation.

SOURCE: Photograph courtesy of the University of Minnesota Archives, University of Minnesota—Twin Cities.

The Minnesota Project (1954–1962) and Surgical Specialization: Medicine as Social Relief or as Biomedical Research?

When the Minnesota Project first began its operations in 1954, its ambitions were quite modest. With faculty members from several universities returning to Seoul in the spring of 1954, buildings that had gone neglected for a period of more than three years from 1950 to 1954 needed to be prepared for the resumption of scholarly activity.[22] Moreover, South Korea had by that point taken on much greater significance in the estimation of America and its international partners, granted the status of "Freedom's Frontier," a potential showcase of "Free World" models and practices bordering on the Communist world, making it an ideal target for the ambitions of both domestic and international reformers.[23] The former governor of Minnesota, Harold Stassen, had succeeded in securing funds as head of FOA (Foreign Operations Administration), the predecessor agency to ICA, and he steered these considerable resources to the benefit of his home state's flagship campus, creating the basis for a lengthy relationship between Minneapolis and Seoul.[24]

On the Seoul end, the South Korean government needed to determine how the funds would be distributed, and there was considerable debate about the possibility of reaching a wider range of recipients. This option was favored by university heads like Paik Nak-Jun (1895–1985) of Yonhi College, who argued that individual institutions should receive resources according to their relative strengths and specific areas of expertise.[25] This design would promote a collectivity among South Korean institutions of higher learning; after all, a similar type of ethic had prevailed during the preceding four years (from 1950 to 1954), with a university collective formed in Pusan managing to sustain a semblance of higher education throughout the war years.[26] Others favored a tight concentration of the funds, with Seoul National University arguing that it merited the majority of the resources as the nation's leading school. Graduates of the university, it argued, would move on to take positions at other institutions, thereby providing a dispersal of any knowledge gained through hosting the original program.[27]

For its part, the University of Minnesota experienced numerous start-up problems with the project, particularly in terms of mobilizing the benefits of the program among its own faculty members. For the engineering program, junior tenure-track faculty expressed great reluctance over the prospect of a one- or two-year assignment to Seoul, a remote and impoverished location at which they were likely to be unable to continue their research.[28] The university eventually had to solicit the participation of external faculty drawn from other universities, with the program to be directed by an external consultant, William Weems, recruited from MIT.[29] Although this design went against the very spirit of ICA guidelines, which emphasized a one-to-one correspondence between a country-specific program and a selected foreign institution, it proved to be a suitable alternative for engineering. Even as 1954 marked the official start of the overall project, little was accomplished in the 1954–1955 period, other than initial site visits made by prominent members of the university hierarchy.

Given this modest beginning, the Minnesota actors conceived of the medical program more as a relief effort than an attempt to offer anything new. That change came only later, introduced under the unique conditions and opportunities provided by the hospital environment. For the first several years of the program, from 1954 to 1957, the emphasis rested primarily on Minneapolis, where visiting doctors and nurses came for clinical study tours, with some of these periods lasting up to two years. This focus also provided sufficient time for the physical rehabilitation of the Seoul facility, which had fallen into disrepair. By 1958, the shift to Seoul began, with pedagogy and clinical practice taking center stage. Returning students from the Minneapolis site trained their peers, and this effort was overseen by a rotating series of visiting personnel from Minnesota, doctors who had volunteered to give the benefit of their time and experience.[30]

For Drs. Lee Chan-Bum and Lee Young-Gyun, the key to the program was based on their close personal relationship, with this bond also contingent on a pair of American mentors: Dr. Walt Lillehei, an internationally renowned cardiac surgeon based at the Minneapolis campus, and Dr. George Schimert (1918–2000), a young surgeon who came to Seoul as part of the exchange, spending approximately a year (1958–1959) developing a chest surgery program and performing numerous demonstration procedures.[31] It was Dr. Schimert who helped to transform interest in the chest to a cardiac program per se, as he chose to pursue only the most ambitious goals, pushing the boundaries of what was then technically feasible at the Seoul facility.[32] Moreover, Schimert believed that it was possible to establish a direct equivalence between Seoul and a comparable American hospital facility, if only the material conditions and training were roughly the same. In pursuit of this aim, he not only lobbied for better equipment at the site but also participated directly in the activities of several Korean professional organizations.

By joining these local meetings, Dr. Schimert made the decision to take the surgical specialization program at Seoul National University into new territory, attempting to teach the latest techniques in heart surgery with almost no intervening period for adjustment. Normally the development of a new procedure requires substantial time before it moves to different sites, with this interval allowing for the purchase of new equipment as well as an extensive training period for staff members to familiarize themselves with new protocols. In contrast, Schimert proposed that the mobilization of the most recent American methods would best serve the interests of the medical program in Seoul and began demonstrating a set of procedures that he had only recently learned during his own residency in Minneapolis. Schimert's self-confidence, along with the trust he placed in his Korean counterparts, Dr. Lee Chan-Bum and Dr. Lee Young-Gyun, was sufficient to justify the radical step he was taking. No longer would the pursuit of thoracic surgery in Seoul imply chest surgery alone; soon it involved complex heart procedures comparable to those being worked out almost simultaneously in the United States.

Under the circumstances, the pool of heart patients at Seoul National University hospital comprised an experimental group in a very real sense, as the types of procedures they underwent involved considerable risk. Under Japanese colonial health, Japanese doctors had policed the health of their colonial subjects on a restricted basis, with the vast majority of Koreans continuing to rely on traditional practitioners to meet the basic necessities of health care.[33] In part because of these lingering associations, the hospital continued to carry with it a set of negative connotations; more importantly, it was not always easy to be admitted, as resources were scarce following the Korean War.[34] The Minnesota Project brought with it not only a program of professionalization but the wholesale transformation of the hospital as a space, a site for biomedical research, with the body of the patient rapidly becoming redefined as an object. By the late 1960s, the hospital possessed a very different identity, and the types of patients and the problems treated each changed in corresponding fashion.

This radical series of transformations also implies a new approach taken with respect to the risks inherent in open-heart surgery. If American institutions underwent a similar transformation at a slightly later point in time, developing the bureaucratic structure of the institutional review board (IRB) to oversee decisions concerning medical research, South Korean hospitals took a different approach at this stage, seeking to control the risk through two means. First, the individual surgeon assumed personal responsibility for maintaining and augmenting his own skills, and we will witness this trope later, as Lee Young-Gyun became a leading figure in South Korean cardiac medicine by the mid-1960s. Second, as a related point, these ambitious surgeons continued their accumulation of new knowledge by forging key relationships with international figures and institutions, linking their own expertise to that of their peers in the course of developing transnational networks.[35] Only through these means could South Korean doctors construct around themselves the appropriate images of authority and skill and, more important, acquire the new technologies they would need to develop surgical expertise.

Mobilizing a Technological Fix: The DeWall Bubble Helix Oxygenator

The confidence with which this overhaul would be executed testifies to the close relationship between the visitors from Minnesota and their South Korean partners, but the overhaul also relied heavily on a technological approach, one that had been developed in Minneapolis earlier in the decade by one of Walt Lillehei's graduate students, Dr. Richard DeWall. Given his interest in the heart, Dr. Lillehei needed to resolve the central issue that had plagued heart surgery from its inception, the difficulty of repairing heart tissue while simultaneously seeking to control the patient's respiration and circulation.[36] The inability to intervene in the heart directly limited most surgical procedures prior to the 1950s to the external portion of the organ, working on the surrounding membrane (pericardium) or possibly with the major (external) vessels responsible for blood flow. Congenital defects inside the heart were almost invariably fatal in children, as there was no means to repair the damaged area without stopping the heart, even when the symptoms were clearly visible via a patient's skin color, typically producing a bluish tinge.[37]

These circumstances would change as the heart group at Minnesota undertook a range of surgeries, carefully building their accumulated skills as a team. Working first with dogs as subjects, and then with human subjects only in carefully selected cases, Dr. Lillehei and his team of residents sought to perfect the techniques associated with cross-circulation, in which a patient volunteered to act as the heart and lungs for a second patient undergoing surgery.[38] With the two subjects connected by a series of tubes, the heart of the volunteer assumed the burden of furnishing the necessary blood supply for two bodies, thereby meeting the needs of the surgical patient. This style of procedure, along with related efforts to regulate and reduce the heart rate through extensive cooling—for example, using an ice bath to slow the heart rate, thereby allowing for temporary intervention—represented the state of the art at the onset of the 1950s, even as the procedure remained enormously risky.[39] Not surprisingly, the volunteer patient was typically a close relative or family member, and frequently the Minnesota team worked with young children, with a parent serving as the volunteer.

The most dramatic change to be associated with this type of procedure came in the mid-1950s with the creation of a set of new technologies that could simulate the action of the human heart. According to a popular version of the story, Richard DeWall, working under Dr. Lillehei as a resident, was relaxing one day after work with a glass of beer. The ascending movement of the bubbles in his glass, rising to the surface, gave DeWall inspiration about a possible means of removing pollutants from the blood, in effect, replicating the actions of the heart and lungs.[40] With plastic tubing and a simple pump, he was able to construct a version of what subsequently came to be known as the bubble helix oxygenator, a device that would transform the possibilities of open-heart surgery. To put it briefly, DeWall's creation safely removed blood from the body with a length of tubing, allowing it to pass through a plastic reservoir following the introduction of fresh oxygen. The blood then passed through a further set of tubes—this length of plastic forming a coil or "helix"—to settle the gas before reentering the body, allowing any excess bubbles to escape.

De Wall's creation required a gradual process of integration into the surgical setting, but, for the first time, the surgeon would have sufficient time to work directly with the tissue of the heart's interior. Moreover, if the helix oxygenator functioned as the equivalent of the lungs, a SigmaMotor pump, a device common to the dairy and brewing industries in Minnesota, functioned as its counterpart, serving as the "heart."[41] The SigmaMotor had long been used for industrial purposes, capable of pumping liquids at a consistent rate and pressure, and it therefore served as an ideal complement to the oxygenator. Later, two SigmaMotor pumps would be employed simultaneously, one each for maintaining the respective arterial and venous blood supplies, making what had been a surgical venture filled with risk into a well-regulated procedure guided by a menu of precise instructions.[42] When the transfer of this technology began to move from Minneapolis to other hospital sites, the SigmaMotor pump became famous in its own right, even as it remained the single most expensive item in the entire surgical package developed at Minnesota.

Together, the bubble helix oxygenator ("lungs") and the SigmaMotor pump ("heart") offered an appealing package, both in terms of their potential ease of use in other settings and, more important, in terms of their transportability. While the pump cost several hundred dollars alone—a cost that could often be met through an outright donation by a partner institution—the remaining components, consisting primarily of a few lengths of plastic tubing, were generally cheap and easily available.[43] With the American research university community acting as the center of a developing network for the export and transfer of these new forms of knowledge and related technologies, the University of Minnesota became one of the leading centers for open-heart surgery and new research into heart technologies during the second half of the 1950s.[44] South Korean participation in the Minnesota Project therefore provided access not simply to the basic elements needed for health care reform (chest surgery, tuberculosis) but also to the latest, cutting-edge forms of American surgical practice.

The arrival of this new technology in Seoul in 1958 explains in large part Dr. Schimert's enthusiasm and desire to participate in the activities of the South Korean medical community. A recent immigrant to the United States following World War II, Schimert had only just completed his own surgical residency under Dr. Lillehei and Dr. Owen Wangensteen (1898–1981), head of surgery at Minnesota, and hoped to make a name for himself on assuming his first position of authority.[45] As for his South Korean partners, Dr. Lee Chan-Bum did not work with Dr. Lillehei, as he had an existing affiliation with the V.A. hospital in Minneapolis, but Lee Young-Gyun had become one of the many foreign residents to train during a residency with Lillehei. This combination of personal experience and firsthand participation on the one hand, along with the cumulative experience of the pair of South Korean doctors on the other, made for a well-matched surgical team, one that would bring this form of emerging practice to Seoul early in the following decade.

At the same time, the complex politics and numerous problems associated with bringing the technology to Seoul will inform the remainder of this chapter, as the hospital facility in Seoul represented a material and professional space quite distinct from that of its counterpart in Minneapolis. If the combination of the bubble helix oxygenator and SigmaMotor pump worked well by the late 1950s, the American success story followed a legacy of failure earlier in the decade. Working first with animals and then with more conservative techniques like cross-circulation, Dr. Lillehei had reached the achievement of open heart surgery only by carefully testing the boundaries of his skills and the capabilities of his equipment.[46] The same objects, when relocated to Seoul in 1958, seldom functioned as expected, as they were embedded within a set of material and social relations specific to the hospital environment of Minneapolis. Instead of rapid success, Drs. Lee Chan-Bum and Lee Young-Gyun encountered great personal frustration, as the vast majority of their patients did not survive the difficult surgery.[47] As they trained the members of their

Seouldae team, crafting a narrative of collective effort, they sought to understand how and why the technological objects functioned differently from their expectations.

Mobilizing Technology in a New Setting: Dr. Schimert and the Demonstration Surgeries of 1958–1959

The process of "technology transfer" to Seoul began with Dr. Schimert's arrival in 1958, the latest among a series of American visitors to assist with the rehabilitation of the medical program at SNU hospital.[48] As a young resident who had worked directly under Dr. Lillehei, moreover, Schimert represented a valuable addition to the project, as he possessed familiarity with the most up-to-date forms of clinical practice. With a commission to start a chest surgery practice at SNU, Schimert arrived full of ambition, eager to test himself in a new environment where he could rely on his own authority in terms of making decisions.[49] Prior to departing for Seoul, however, Schimert had expressed reluctance to commit to the South Korean project, fearing that it might delay his career ambitions, especially his desire to secure a position as a surgeon at a leading American facility.[50] His advisors at Minnesota, Dr. Owen Wangensteen in particular, had persuaded him that the overseas experience in an unfamiliar context would offer a suitable test of his leadership potential.[51]

His reluctance to commit to Seoul is critical in understanding Schimert's subsequent use of the context as his research base, as arguably he would push the boundaries of his commission to stretch the limits of the original agreement, a mission to start a thoracic surgery and cardiac catheterization unit.[52] Prior to his departure, Schimert had informed Dean Diehl (1891–1973) of the University of Minnesota Medical School about his concern that a leave of absence for the academic year 1957–1958 might delay his graduation, only to be reassured that the work would "constitute an invaluable experience for a person interested in an academic career in the future."[53] To ensure that the rhetorical force of his remarks was clear, Diehl clarified these remarks by adding that "I personally would feel able to give a stronger recommendation . . . to a person with a broad background of experience of this type."[54] Dr. Schimert, who had made a tentative commitment to the project earlier in his residency, now found himself pressured to accept the position in Seoul, knowing that this choice coincided precisely with his superior's wishes.

This period of doubt on Schimert's part, even if it soon yielded to pragmatic considerations, plays a critical role in understanding him both as an individual along with his newfound enthusiasm for cardiac surgery in Seoul. Moreover, Dean Diehl was not alone in expressing his views to Schimert, as Dr. Wangensteen also emphasized to his younger colleague the necessity of committing to the South Korea project. Wangensteen, who privately characterized Schimert as a "venturesome" young surgeon, felt that the experience would prove formative, offering an opportunity for significant growth and maturation both as a person and a surgeon.[55] Known more for his enthusiasm with research and new technologies, Schimert would gain the benefit of interacting with and supervising a large number of personnel in a new setting, a developmental experience that could not easily be replicated in the American context.

This possibility explains Schimert's subsequent decision to use the setting as the base for much of his own research, continuing a trend from his residency at Minnesota, where he had designed his own version of an oxygenator.[56] In Seoul, Schimert did everything possible to standardize the elements of cardiac care, building on the new regimen of clinical rotations that had started one year prior to his arrival (1957–1959). Rather than adopting a conservative approach based on the limited material resources, he took the opposite stance, viewing the hospital as analogous to a blank template, a space on which he might imprint his vision.

By the time of his arrival in July 1958, moreover, the SNU hospital site had already undergone substantial renovation, making for greater research possibilities in the new context. A total of forty SNU staff members had traveled to Minnesota for training in the preceding years (from 1954 to 1957), with thirty-eight of these individuals returning to resume their positions.[57] Unlike his immediate predecessors, Schimert did not need to spend significant time bringing the program up to speed, so the majority of his time could be devoted to the teaching and practice of clinical medicine. With a commission to teach the most recent techniques and practices, Schimert decided to provide a number of demonstration procedures, working side by side with South Korean doctors in the operating room. This activity stood as a practical lesson in observation and also permitted hands-on participation for a limited number of selected Korean colleagues.

As for these participants, Schimert developed close relationships with students and colleagues at SNU, and he took care to promote their work whenever presented with an opportunity. In the report he submitted to University of Minnesota on completion of his overseas tour, he noted specifically the capabilities of this community, with surgeons performing difficult procedures "with more skill than when similar operations are performed by the average Western physician."[58] He exhibited a similar level of confidence in the equipment he brought to the context, noting the potential of the bubble helix oxygenator and its related components: "The development of safe extracorporeal circulation and its introduction into routine clinical use . . . [has] finally made it possible to perform operations inside of the heart under direct vision."[59] For Schimert, the procedure he transfered to Seoul was a finished product in every respect, consisting of a menu of instructions for the surgeon to follow and a set of reliable, mechanical components to assist him with the task.

Again, Schimert's commission on departure for Seoul had consisted of a chest surgery practice, and the transition he made to adapt this mission into performing open-heart surgery represented a significant move forward in terms of removing a series of intermediate steps. At Minnesota, work with the helix oxygenator began only after a lengthy series of trials, first with animals and then with human subjects, working under carefully controlled conditions.[60] Expressing confidence in his own abilities as a teacher and confident in the reliability of his equipment, Schimert saw the major challenge in Seoul to be enforcing a consistent pedagogy and standardization, twin goals that should overcome any material or cultural differences between the two settings. On an implicit level, he embraced a doctrine of equivalence, a belief that the hospital site in Seoul held no major differences from his prior experience with his patients in Minnesota.

Along with the surgical procedure itself, Schimert's belief in standardization took precedence as one of the major teaching points, especially with respect to the pre- and postoperative care of heart patients. At Minnesota, Dr. Lillehei, while not yet subject to oversight from an IRB, had consulted carefully with his colleagues before selecting prospective subjects, weighing their opportunities for survival. Making this decision in conjunction with Dr. Owen Wangensteen, Lillehei ultimately selected a target group consisting largely of young patients, those born with congenital heart defects—typically a defect in the septum separating the heart's chambers.[61] This type of procedure became his preferred procedure in the course of perfecting the surgery, and it did not hurt that the recovery stages made for excellent publicity images when these young candidates returned to good health.[62]

Likewise, Schimert sought to bring this kind of careful scrutiny to Seoul, and he had a pool of potential patients with lung and heart problems from which to select. Moreover, he recognized that postoperative care was absolutely critical in these cases, particularly in the days immediately following surgery. Dr. Schimert therefore brought a routinized approach to bear on the problem, requesting regular checks on a patient's condition to monitor physical well-being. Prior to 1958, Korean surgeons had had very limited experience in working with the heart, with common procedures restricted to the removal of lung tissue or pericardiectomy, removal of part of the membrane surrounding the heart.[63] Schimert pushed beyond this knowledge to new areas, attempting to teach both the actual procedure and its follow-up forms of care in terms of a menu of instructions, a set of rules that could be easily replicated, thereby minimizing the element of risk.

Moreover, this part of Schimert's approach was entirely in keeping with the ethic of pedagogical reform then taking shape at the hospital. As noted earlier, the introduction of new professional categories coincided with a critical period (1957–1959) in which three new professional categories were integrated at one–year intervals. This measure not only transformed the focus on clinical practice and anatomy at the hospital but, more important, began to break down the hierarchical authority of senior personnel: New residents and interns in training would begin to do much of the actual hands-on work, with clinical rounds conducted on a daily basis. From the perspective of heart surgery, the rigorous regime of postoperative care, requiring a schedule of constant monitoring, would suit the new demands placed on residents and interns. If Schimert's goals were radical, his methods remained fairly conventional in terms of execution, as he worked within the framework of both the hospital and the social expectations of the local medical community.

Within the modest span of slightly more than a year (1958–1959), Schimert managed to perform an estimated thirty demonstration procedures, covering the entire range of chest surgeries that he could expect to be valuable to his South Korean peers.[64] Given his aim of establishing a cardiac program, the surgeries included at least one open-heart surgery, with Lee Chang Bum among those able to assist, prior to his departure for the Minneapolis VA hospital. Although Lee Young-Gyun was absent from Seoul during much of this time, his residency nonetheless allowed him to experience direct supervision under Walt Lillehei, this being more than ample compensation. Moreover, Lee Young-Gyun was one of the Minnesota Project participants fortunate enough to receive a second year of training, as his advisors felt that the additional time would do him good. By the beginning of the 1960s, the two Korean physicians returned to Seoul to begin work together, where they would begin assembling the elements of a South Korean thoracic surgery team, attempting to replicate the procedures on their own.

"All of My Patients are Dying": Facing Challenges in Assembling a Thoracic Surgery Team (1961–1968)

With the combined experience of the two surgeons, Seoul National University Hospital believed that it had the necessary elements to begin assembling its own heart surgery team, training additional support personnel according to the new clinical regime. Although the formal relationship with Minnesota ended in June 1962—against Minnesota's will, the Seoul side permitted the contract to lapse—the relationship between Dr. Lillehei and Lee Young-Gyun, his former student, continued to flourish over the next several decades.[65] As both Drs. Lee had already participated in the work of open-heart surgery, the pair were confident that they could integrate the DeWall bubble helix technology, along with its corresponding support mechanisms, in the process of implementing the surgical procedures in the Seoul context. What the two men underestimated was the extent to which both the imported technology and the surgery itself were embedded in the social context of Minneapolis, particularly the social relations present within an urban hospital setting.

If Dr. Schimert had presented the new pedagogy he brought in 1958 as essentially a complete set of instructions, he also did everything possible to establish a doctrine of equivalence between the UMN Hospital and the comparable facilities he had visited in Seoul. More important, Schimert's confidence in this assumption was shared by his South Korean counterparts, who were eager to begin the chore of mastering the difficult surgery on their own terms. Less than three years after Schimert's departure, Dr. Lee Chan-Bum was leading a number of procedures designed to familiarize members of his team with the new work of performing heart surgery.[66] Even as he had hoped to accelerate the pace of the learning curve, Dr. Lee recognized the need to work with animals first as a valuable form of preparation, before moving on to work with human subjects, a much riskier proposition.[67]

Prior to considering the range of surgical procedures attempted by the pair of surgeons, it is worth recalling the circumstances on which they based much of this work. The new professional categories (clerk, intern, resident) introduced during the Minnesota Project were still very much in flux in 1962, meaning that South Korean health care professionals did not necessarily have

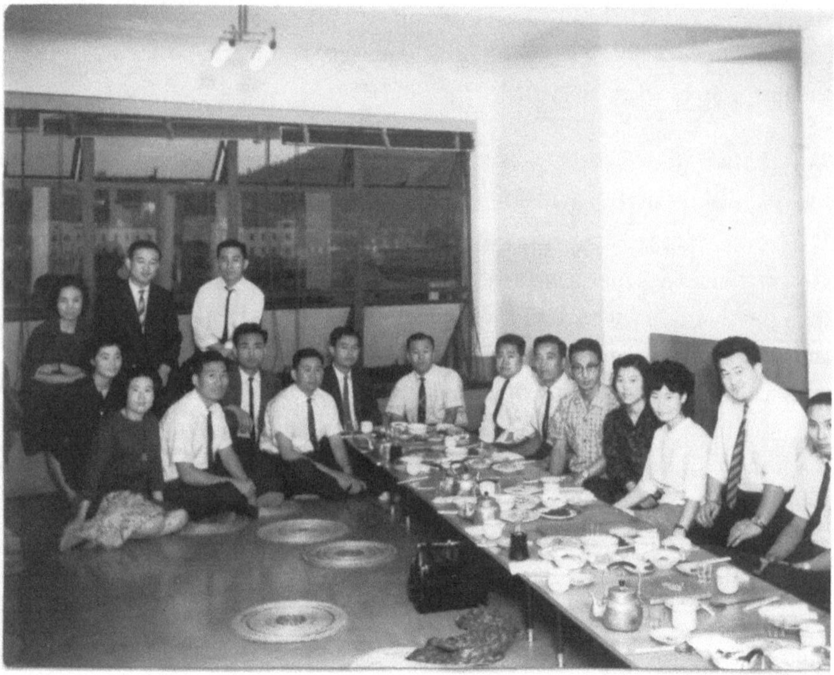

Members of the growing "heart community" at Seoul National University Hospital share a meal in a 1965. Dr. Lee Young-Gyun sits fifth from the right, with Dr. Lee Chan-Bum to his right.

Source: Kim Won-gon, SNU Hospital.

a firm sense of the individual responsibilities assigned within the operating theater. To put this in other terms, the *chogyo*, or assistants, typically needed to assume responsibility for multiple tasks in the operating room (OR) during surgery.[68] This practice held significant implications for new surgical specialties, as the critical job of the anesthesiologist, for example, had not even been created yet, or certainly not as an exclusive responsibility. In practice, this meant that much of the technical learning, the process of familiarization, was done on the job, with support personnel facing a steep learning curve while learning alongside the supervising surgeon.

At the material level as well, the hospital in Seoul represented a very different type of space in comparison with its American counterpart. Although Dr. Lillehei had succeeded in Minneapolis, he achieved his aims only by training a close-knit group of surgeons and support personnel together over a period lasting more than a decade. In the case of SNU, this experience factor became especially problematic due to the lack of support personnel—in terms of both their numbers and previous professional training. The need for constant monitoring of heart patients, especially in the postoperative phases, placed severe stress on the capabilities of the existing system. Even as the technology represented an apparent quick fix to the central problem of transferring the surgical protocol, basic material issues cropped up frequently, undercutting the effectiveness of the new training and equipment.

Materiality and the South Korean Hospital

The limited resources of the hospital site made SNU Hospital, along with its peer institutions in South Korea, a very different kind of space in the early 1960s. Families were permitted, and in fact encouraged, to assume the task of feeding and caring for a family member who was a patient, meaning that there was little formality in terms of establishing, let alone enforcing, a common practice such as visiting hours.[69] This lack of professional distinction carried over to the work of assessment, with few resources available for the evaluation of tissue samples and biological specimens on site. Under the circumstances, the hospital's priority lay with the diagnosis and treatment of those patients deemed to have an acute need, rather than with adopting a policy of open admission. In this sense, it could be difficult to get admitted to a hospital, as the availability of a bed and the prospect of responding to treatment had to be weighed carefully. At a very basic level, hospital practice intersected heavily with the everyday world of family life, despite claims to the contrary.

These issues would in turn shape the patient base on which the entire surgical procedure depended. Whereas in Minnesota Dr. Lillehei had carefully selected from among a roster of young patients, those likely to represent ideal candidates for survival, Drs. Lee Chan-Bum and Lee Young-Gyun had no such luxury when they began their work with human subjects. In Seoul, the typical client was likely to be a bit older, possibly even approaching middle age, and the damage to be repaired included not only a range of congenital heart defects but also a wide range of problems typically associated with lifestyle choices (for example, diet or smoking).[70] Of the first twenty patients to undergo some version of the open heart surgery in Korea (dating from 1963), five were more than thirty years old, with another five in their twenties.[71] The age range spanned from those with congenital defects, the youngest at the age of four, to one patient in his early fifties, with this wide range suggesting that the South Korean doctors needed to be far more liberal in determining suitable candidates.[72]

Moreover, this change to the process led to complex personal negotiations going into the surgery. With no formal set of regulations governing the choice, the South Korean doctors could only offer their counsel to the patients they encountered, hoping that at least a few would consent to undergo the surgery. Given the attending risks, only those experiencing great pain or expecting imminent death were likely to make such a choice. Not surprisingly, one of the most common problems typifying this first group of subjects was tetralogy of Fallot (TOF), in which there is low oxygenation of the blood ("blue baby") caused by abnormalities in the heart.[73] In terms of their results, the surgeons found the task of maintaining respiration and circulation during surgery was eased by the bubble helix technology, but this alone was not enough to ensure success. The pace of the learning curve for the surgery began to decelerate early in the decade of the 1960s as the South Korean team experienced a number of setbacks, with their patients typically expiring during surgery or shortly after.

Dr. Lee Young-Gyun experienced this development as a moment of personal doubt, assuming responsibility for his failure to achieve better results in the operating theatre. Writing to his mentor, Dr. Lillihei, in 1965, he observed that "all of my patients are dying," a poignant remark that offered little context, even as it did not seek refuge in alternative explanations.[74] Instead, Dr. Lee sought to transform the situation through sheer hard work and effort, requesting permission to return to the United States for a second study tour during the second half of the 1960s. In his estimation, the solution lay with a refresher course involving direct participation in cardiac surgery in the United States, where he would reacquaint himself with the particulars through observation. The knowledge necessary to resolve the current impasse, whether in tacit or explicit form, was understood to inhabit the material space of the operating room in Minneapolis and equally in the comforting presence of Dr. Lillihei, his senior mentor and teacher.

Before turning to the critical issue of establishing local control over the OR, the retrospective justification for pursuing a program of heart surgery from the perspective of the South Korean actors deserves mention here, as we have already looked briefly at Dr. Schimert's reasoning. Many official accounts in Korean now cite the decision as one of pursuing a systemic rationale, that is, to choose those specific skill areas that allowed for the training of an entire surgical team as a unit.[75] This explanation makes sense for clinical medicine as a whole and even with the decision to pursue new surgeries of a limited scope, but it cannot account for heart surgery per se, a risky procedure regardless of the site and especially so in the South Korean context. These accounts tend to factor in developments taking place at nearby institutions, with doctors at Severance Hospital offering competition in cardiac care and with the National Medical Center putting together its own comprehensive program of medical rehabilitation (1958–1968). Again, even as this systemic claim offers a convenient rationale in retrospect, it cannot encompass the scope of Schimert's ambitions, nor does it anticipate the many difficult experiences that the Korean surgeons would soon encounter.

Establishing Open-Heart Surgery in Seoul (1961–1964)

A New Type of Surgeon?

In leaving behind a conspicuous paper trail through his presence in Seoul and Minneapolis, Dr. Lee Young-Gyun provides ample evidence that Dr. Schimert was not the only one with professional ambitions, and the scope of his subsequent career supports this observation. Prior to returning to Seoul (1959), the young surgeon lobbied University of Minnesota authorities for the privilege of participating in heart surgery, noting that the "official application blanks were filled and signed in Korea for this specific CV [cardiovascular] training."[76] This open appeal to bureaucratic procedure might not be enough, though, so Dr. Lee made sure to mobilize a larger set of humanitarian concerns, adding that the "CV surgery field was chosen for me as the policy of the school in Seoul by my department chief and the dean."[77] With this logic bolstering his rationale, Dr. Lee awaited permission to begin the final stages of his clinical training in heart surgery.

Before making this appeal, he had already undergone extensive preparation at Minneapolis in a variety of clinical settings, beginning with an initial period of five months on "red and white service," followed by eight months working in Dr. Lillehei's experimental dog lab, where much of the new heart work was still being tested and perfected on animals.[78] Following this familiarization period of slightly more than a year, Dr. Lee moved on to working specifically with human anatomy, with a two-month clinical rotation assigned to the cardiac catheterization lab and then a subsequent two months assigned directly to Dr. Lillehei's supervision within his diagnostic section.[79] Even as this training suggests a clear pattern, preparing the trainee for future work with the new surgery, Dr. Lee's anxiety became palpable, as he feared that he might miss a critical opportunity. His letter outlining his request in

February 1959 captures this tension, emphasizing that he had been "waiting and prepared for this [new clinical training] for one and a half years."[80]

In case there were any doubts about his aims, he noted an "earnest desire to follow Dr. Schimrt's [sic] open heart or start it," underscoring his interest in building an independent heart program in Seoul. Even more so than his close colleague, Lee Chan-Bum, the ambitious Lee Young-Gyun recognized the potential value of this work in terms of opening up career opportunities, although he carefully framed his ambitions in humanistic terms, the possibility of bringing this work to "a far away country, Korea for the benefit of my country people, my school."[81] Moreover, he reassured his superiors in Minneapolis about the preparations then being made in Seoul, covering the fields relevant to implementing a new surgical program, including "x-ray, cardiology, pediatric cardiology, [and] anesthesiology."[82] Most important, much of the necessary expertise overlapped with the interests of the Minnesota Project, and Dr. Lee was quick to note the names of his (Korean) colleagues who had prepared for these critical areas.

Both in his rhetoric and his appeals to the theme of (site) equivalence, Dr. Lee constructed a case comparable to the one previously made by Dr. Schimert in his own account of developments taking place in Seoul, circa 1958–1959. However, even more so than Dr. Schimert, a short-term visitor, Dr. Lee had to be familiar with the problem of material deficiencies in Seoul, and indeed he soon began to write letters on a regular basis requesting basic supplies from his close friends and American colleagues. This is not to suggest that he misrepresented the extent of preparations at the SNU hospital facility, but certainly Dr. Lee chose to portray these events highly selectively and with a strong degree of optimism, emphasizing both the potential of the heart program and its value for professional development. Only when he returned to Seoul was he confronted with the material realities of his circumstances, in which the available patients were few and the hospital support system was sorely lacking.

The Patient Population at SNU Hospital (1961–1964)

To recall a point made previously, the patient population at Minnesota was generally determined by a preliminary consultation between Drs. Lillehei and Wangensteen, occupying their respective roles as head of the heart program and chief of surgery, with Dr. Wangensteen carefully weighing his junior colleague's requests. In the absence of a review board or a similar form of oversight, the two doctors considered factors such as the age of a patient, his or her present condition, and, most important, the likelihood of survival. In contrast, Dr. Lee Young-Gyun had no such luxury in Seoul and in fact complained about the moderate pace of his program, observing in 1961 that he "would like to go faster, things in Korea move rather slowly."[83] This remark has to be placed in the context of his pool of available subjects, which was rather limited, leaving Dr. Lee to note that "I am very unhappy that only risky and difficult cases are available for a beginner like me."[84]

Under ideal conditions, Dr. Lee would have chosen to work almost exclusively with a patient group similar to that to which he had been exposed to in Minneapolis, selecting carefully from among the best cases to perform surgery on those (young) candidates likely to thrive under a careful inspection regime of postoperative care. In practical terms, this generally meant a group of young children, those born with congenital heart defects that could be repaired, at least in part. Although such cases—including a range of ASD (atrial septal defect) and VSD (ventricular septal defect) cases, along with tetralogy of Fallot—remained problematic in the early 1960s, Dr. Lillehei's team had begun to experience a high degree of success; again, the relative youth and health of these patients boded well for their subsequent period of recovery.[85] Given his familiarity with such cases, it is reasonable to speculate that this description approximates what Dr. Lee might have envisioned had circumstances been different.

In terms of the constraints these circumstances placed on the nascent heart program, this meant that the South Korean team could proceed only at great risk, and at a highly reduced pace, averaging approximately one new case a month as of the summer of 1961.[86] For his part, Dr. Lee acknowledged the ethical dilemma in which this placed him, noting his willingness to undertake this difficult work, adding that "if I wait for less risky cases I wouldn't be able to do a case at all for several years at least."[87] To occupy his remaining time, Dr. Lee simultaneously started work with a dog lab, a facility where he could work with animals as a substitute for human subjects, perfecting his surgical technique. This work, too, represented an approximation of his experience in Minnesota, albeit in a somewhat accelerated version, and here Dr. Lee was able to practice at least several times a week, keeping his skills sharp while waiting for the next patient to appear.

To this point, Lee Young-Gyun was sustained largely by his enthusiasm and eagerness to develop an independent heart program, and only over the next several years (from 1962 through 1965) did cumulative difficulties begin to erode his confidence. Two observations are in order here, both with respect to the developing relationship between the program in Minneapolis and its partner group in Seoul. First, Dr. Lee recognized the material differences on returning home almost immediately, and, although he refused to cite this factor as the major source of his problems, it appeared in his letters to Dr. Lillehei over the next several years as a recurring theme. Second, Dr. Lee maintained an awareness of his patients as individual subjects, and this is not surprising as he began to put a full-scale research program into place. This is not to suggest that he would become hardened or callous in the near future but, again, to emphasize the relative novelty of conducting this brand of newer biomedical research in South Korea.

In a recovering nation with a limited number of available beds, hospital admissions represented a tricky business, with a general policy of admitting only the most acute cases. At the same time, this limited number of beds was frequently not in (full) use, as hospitals continued to carry negative associations. Dr. Lee Young-Gyun's emerging research program, conducted with the assistance of Dr. Lee Chan-Bum and a number of collaborators, ran contrary to this conservative trend, encouraging that patients not only be admitted but that they also receive treatment promptly. The Minnesota Project had specifically encouraged this type of aim, augmenting the pedagogy, the facilities, and the ambitions of the hospital, but these ambitions strained the existing resources of the hospital. In turn, Dr. Lee's frustration over the lack of rapid progress was obvious, particularly as he was required to proceed cautiously according to the pool of available patients.

"Cheap, Inexpensive" Technology: "Technology Transfer" versus the Material Realities

Although Lee Young-Gyun could not question the use of imported technology, he recognized that it presented inherent difficulties, in terms of both familiarization with its use and obtaining replacement parts when the originals developed signs of wear. The visiting Minnesota team had made much of the "transportability" of their surgical package when it first became available (in 1958 through 1961), providing a menu of instructions, substantial pedagogical assistance, and the necessary physical components (bubble oxygenator). This last object in particular was often characterized as "cheap and inexpensive," consisting of a series of plastic tubes and components, reflecting the story of its origins in Dr. DeWall's imaginative rendering. In 1961, however, Dr. Lee discovered that this object did not fit his circumstances in Seoul, nor was he able to obtain the necessary replacement parts, at least certainly not without appealing to the international market. In other words, the very features mobilized as the major selling points of the American technology proved to be highly suspect in the Korean context.

In the case of the SigmaMotor, the firm became best known for its heart pumps during the period immediately following the Korean War, from 1953 through 1967, soon branching out into related forms of technology associated with kidney dialysis.[88] More specifically, the SigmaMotor T-6 was the model used most commonly in Seoul, although the firm would market roughly four different types of pump over the period during which open-heart techniques were being perfected.[89] As noted previously, the expense of the pump, often the single largest cost in terms of transferring the surgery to a new site, was frequently met by a donation of the equipment, as was likely the case with SNU hospital. With its design aimed at preventing corrosion, the T-6 limited contact between its liquid contents—whether blood, as in this case, or corrosive chemicals in industrial uses—and its inner components. This translated into a much longer period of use, leaving ample time to become familiar with the device and its technical specifications. The major replacements required for maintenance involved the lengths of plastic tubing, essential for conveying liquids, and, in the case of heart surgery, absolutely critical to maintaining a safe, sterile environment.

Even with such a simple procedure, the replacement of lengths of plastic tubing would create major difficulties in Seoul, a site where the reliable manufacture of industrial plastics based on petrochemicals did not take place domestically until at least the late 1960s or early 1970s.[90] For the heart surgeon, this meant that two activities typically took place simultaneously: Lengths of tubing from abroad had to be hoarded and extended to their maximum period of use, while the surgeon also had to make regular appeals to colleagues and friends for additional supplies of such materials. In the case of Dr. Lee Young-Gyun, his letters from the early to mid-1960s are filled with such requests, when he regularly consulted with his former advisor (Lillehei) for technical assistance. In July 1963, for example, Dr. Lee wrote that "I am cleaning my used helix major tube with great intention but not without reluctance," an act presumably undertaken in anticipation of an upcoming surgical case.[91] The language here reinforces the difficulties faced in surgery, while hinting at the problem of material deficiencies, underscoring the need for better equipment without necessarily making a direct appeal.

In other cases, Dr. Lee felt it necessary to address his needs explicitly, and the program of exchange between Minnesota and Seoul continued well beyond the initial period covered under the terms of the ICA contract, from 1954 through 1962). The basic elements of heart surgery—supplies and component parts associated with the procedure itself, along with the elements comprising follow-up care—represented a major issue in Seoul, as these essentials proved unavailable on the local market. The most commonly used anticoagulant, heparin solution, was another such item, and Dr. Lee frequently requested samples of the sponges commonly used in surgery, Ivalon, along with component parts for working with the mitral valve.[92] A procedure far from perfected in the early 1960s, open-heart surgery required active participation in an emerging transnational network of exchange, forcing the South Korean surgeons to depend on their American colleagues at a time when the acquisition of even basic medical supplies proved beyond their means.

To briefly illustrate the importance of this type of exchange, heparin had been first introduced about two decades earlier, in the late 1930s, to limit pulmonary embolism and vein thrombosis in the course of working with the heart.[93] In its clinical usage, it became especially valuable in the postoperative context, aiding when a patient was at the most vulnerable stages of his or her recovery. Similarly, the Ivalon (polyvinyl) sponge served as one of the most commonly used tools in the repair of heart defects, typically functioning as filler material to "patch" a hole or breach within the surrounding tissue. The types of septal defects commonly treated by heart surgeons at this time, ASD and VSD, required the use of such materials in substantial quantities. Without the Ivalon and heparin, Dr. Lee could still proceed, but effectively he was functioning without a full complement of tools, a factor that no doubt affected his criteria for selection of patients and the reduced pace of surgical work in Seoul.

The creation of new supply chains between partner nations (United States, South Korea) following a lengthy period of pedagogical exchange should not appear to be anything more than it is, an expected development given the circumstances. At the same time, its absence from much of the literature reinforces the reduced character of "technology transfer," the Cold War rhetoric in which a fixed object or technological system moves from point A to point B, assuming the stability of the technology in question and a near equivalence between two sites in material terms.[94] Again, the hospital in Seoul represented a distinct space in which the performance of the open-heart procedure had to be reworked, "translated" to meet a new set of conditions and skill requirements. Moreover, the creation of this supply chain underscores a conspicuous power difference, requiring that South Korean surgeons join new international forms of exchange. In brief, the teaching of the procedure was not so much a matter of pedagogy as an issue of eliciting South Korean participation in an emerging transnational network of biomedicine.[95]

Prior to his encounter with the Minnesota Project, Lee Young-Gyun would have encountered new colleagues almost exclusively within northeast Asia (Korea, Japan), even as the Korean War brought an increasing number of American medical personnel to the peninsula. This transition should not be taken lightly, as the experience of new models and pedagogy would radically transform the practice and possibilities available to South Korean surgeons. Moreover, Lee Young-Gyun soon mobilized his relationships with Americans to enter other international medical networks, studying in Sweden from 1965 to 1966. The word *relationship* remains key here, as the ambitions of ROK state planners ultimately had to be grounded in the dynamics of personal connections, quite often contingent on a relationship between a mentor and his or her former student.

Reinforcing this point, Dr. Lillehei became an eager collaborator with his former student, helping him to resolve both the material and surgical difficulties outlined here. By 1963, their letters bear signs of a relationship developing between peers—evident in both the content and the form of address used—and Dr. Lillehei felt comfortable in advising a slower pace for the Korean program, not because he held a low estimation of its potential but largely because of these material issues. The surgeries that Lee Young-Gyun hoped to attempt required the use of prosthetic heart valves, an item that could be supplied only at irregular intervals. With his ambitions and an increasing caseload straining his resources, Dr. Lee had not yet achieved surgical success, but he would do so very soon; in the process, he was rapidly changing his surgical practice and personal identity within Korean medical circles.

Perhaps most important, Dr. Lee linked these two critical issues—the role of patient intake and the availability of surgical materials—by consciously mobilizing the notion of paying clients as a future goal, even more so than surgical success itself. Achieving surgical success implies that paying clients would likely find their way to the hospital, aware of the possibility of an extended life span, but for Lee, the two were intertwined in terms of subsidizing the material basis for the surgery itself. In a May 1963 letter to Walt Lillehei, he noted that "either [sic] I nor the hospital can replace the expendable parts of the oxygenator," a development he attributed to a pool of "charity patients who pay nothing at all to the hospital," leaving his program with little room for growth.[96] Dr. Lee subsequently closed this same letter by outlining his future plans, adding that "I imagine it will take a little more time till I can have paying patients."[97]

Mobilizing "Thoracic Surgery" at SNU (1965–1968): Strengthening Networks of Exchange

Traced through his private correspondence, Dr. Lee's approach to the possibility of subsidizing a higher standard of health care by attracting a patient base was framed in terms of a lengthy period of personal sacrifice, after which he planned to enter another form of practice. He hinted at this ambition frequently, openly acknowledging it to Dr. Lillehei, stating that "my desire is at least some steady results has [sic] to be established in open heart surgery before I quit for a little better personal living for me and my family."[98] What this alternative might have been Dr. Lee never reveals, but presumably he was considering the chance to take his expertise to another setting, possibly relocating outside South Korea.[99] This is important in that the chance of developing a lucrative medical practice was simply unimaginable in South Korea in the decade of the 1960s. South Korea remained a poor, agrarian nation, still experiencing the effects of the recent war, with its ambitions limited to the immediate goals of economic recovery, subsistence, and rehabilitation.

What is fascinating is the extent to which Dr. Lee's personal ambitions would undergo a radical transformation in the next two decades, with economic revitalization transforming the character of South Korean health care dramatically by the mid- to late 1980s. The arrival of a social welfare system—referring here to a national health insurance scheme originating in 1963, conducted on a very limited basis, with subsequent reforms coming in 1977 and 1989—was "late," meaning that citizens were asked to make personal sacrifices for the sake of economic growth, a style of government that has frequently been characterized in the scholarship as a "developmental dictatorship."[100] This summary of the period offers only a limited perspective, though, and it is within the material practices of medicine that we can see the process taking shape. For Lee Young-Gyun and other ambitious surgeons like him, this meant the necessity of mobilizing their research and their career ambitions, even as these were still very much in process: In brief, Dr. Lee served as an advocate for South Korean heart surgery, claiming its readiness, even as his program had yet to achieve any substantive results.

Although SNU hospital did not formally proclaim a thoracic surgery program as such until 1968, its aim was evident from the early 1960s, a tribute to the combined will of the ambitious American visitor, George Schimert, and his main South Korean collaborator, Lee Young-Gyun, who achieved his first tentative success with open heart surgery in 1964. For his part, Dr. Lee Chan-Bum was present for much of the early period of the program, but he passed away in 1967, having dedicated his professional life to developing work in this new area. Lee Young-Gyun in turn became the public face for much of heart surgery, both at the hospital and in his practice, where he was involved in the complex series of steps from limited publicly subsidized health care to a system that later embraced the private clinic with relatively light government regulation by the following decade, the 1990s.

Accumulating Expertise through International Networks? (1965–)

To return to the 1965 context, Lee Young-Gyun remained ambivalent about the fate of the heart surgery program, even as he had marked his first personal success a year earlier.[101] As of August, Lee found himself overwhelmed with work, treating a wide variety of heart cases, ranging from the fairly routine to the acute.[102] As noted previously, the lack of materials represented a persisting problem, forcing him to make frequent requests of partners as he sought to develop a network of suppliers. Related to this effort, Dr. Lee recognized that his relationship with his former adviser, providing valuable clinical experience, could be augmented by seeking a similar role in another context. In late 1965, he therefore traveled to Sweden on a SIDA (Sweden International Cooperation Development Agency) fellowship, a program that provided him with funds to travel and study at Uppsala University for a year, exposing him to the context of thoracic surgery in Europe under the supervision of Dr. Viking Björk (1918–2009).

The August 1965 letter in which Dr. Lee announced this good news to Dr. Lillehei is a remarkable study in contrasts, as the document juxtaposes the fellowship announcement against the twin themes of material deprivation and personal struggle. At times, Dr. Lee borders on despair, noting the numerous failures among his recent cases, including "all eight cyanotic tetrads."[103] He follows this summary with a telling line, assuming personal responsibility for the failed cases, observing that "there must be something wrong with me."[104] As it turns out, we learn that this observation combines genuine emotion with rhetorical strategy, with Dr. Lee framing his remarks carefully. Specifically, the perceived failure provides the context for a request for a return American visit, a "refresher" course of study, either with Lillehei's group or another such group. In seeking to restore his confidence, Dr. Lee sought direct access to a legacy of success, something he had not experienced since departing Minnesota six years earlier. At the same time, he was, consciously or not, adding to his personal network, ensuring that his lines of communication and supplies would no longer pose a problem.

For Lee Young-Gyun, this did not simply represent a trip devoted to further clinical experience—although the Uppsala University hospital would provide him with valuable exposure to a new context—as he had already spent two years in Minneapolis nearly a decade earlier. Rather, it marked recognition that his American contacts alone were not sufficient as a network of suppliers for heart surgery materials, the realization that further expansion of his contacts might prove beneficial both from a personal and a professional standpoint. Beginning in October 1965, Dr. Lee began a nine-month clinical fellowship focusing on "open heart surgery with left heart catheterization," after which he hoped to make a short visit of approximately two to three months to the United States.[105] Moreover, when he announced his plans to Dr. Lillehei, as noted previously, he hinted strongly that he would not mind an invitation to return to Minnesota, nor would he object to any recommendations concerning sources of financial support for the visit.

It is reasonable to speculate that the opportunity to travel to Sweden stemmed from frequent contact with international colleagues at the National Medical Center (Kungnip Ŭiryowŏn) in Seoul, which was staffed largely by doctors from three Scandinavian countries from 1958 through 1968, as they continued their relief work following the Korean War.[106] In addition, the "Dr. Björk" referred to briefly in Lee's letter was himself an extremely prominent heart surgeon, one of the world's leading figures, requiring no further explanation in the letter to Lillehei. Viking Olov Björk had only recently (1962) assumed a position as professor at Upsalla University hospital and, at the time of Lee's clinical fellowship, was just preparing a move to a subsequent position at the Karolinska Institute (1966), where he remained for the rest of his career.[107] Having already achieved the chance to train under the prominent American, Dr. Lillehei, Lee Young-Gyun now sought to develop a personal relationship with one of the leading figures in Europe, knowing that this relationship could enhance his career prospects.

For his part, Dr. Björk, like Dr. Lillehei, sought to develop partnerships with surgeons from other national contexts by encouraging their participation in these clinical fellowships. On this point, the funds provided by SIDA granted Dr. Lee a sum sufficient to travel to Stockholm and live there with little difficulty, although he would lament that he would be unable to save funds due to the relatively high cost of living. Regardless, though, he was pleased to receive the opportunity to work with Dr. Björk, who had a similar background to that of Lee Chan-Bum, beginning first with lung surgery and the effects of tuberculosis.[108] With the move to Uppsala in 1958, moreover, Björk had started his own program in the form of a cardiothoracic unit, beginning his own career as a major innovator. Although the material circumstances were very different in Europe, this context provided Dr. Lee with the chance to observe a heart program at its inception, with training and pedagogical issues of its own.

Dr. Björk's surgical specialty, working with the heart's left ventricle, represented a personal innovation, a development worked out in part through his prior work with the lungs. Specifically, he determined that it was possible to measure pressure in the left side by first inserting a needle through the right posterior chest, before passing it through the left atrium.[109] Along with a catheter, the needle's position allowed for new measurements to be taken, thereby gauging pressure in the left ventricle, the left atrium, and the aorta.[110] For Dr. Lee, the encounter with this new work—also in its developmental stages in the early 1950s—was similar to his rotation through Minnesota, with the added factor that the Upsalla hospital was itself very much a site undergoing transition and, in this respect, much closer to the type of problem familiar to the Koreans. Although Lee was not able to make a second study tour to the United States, his enthusiasm for Sweden is evident, and he then had access to international networks for his supplies.

Although this factor increased his access to supplies, it did not make an immediate difference in terms of the patterns of surgeries he attempted on his return from Sweden in late 1966. Based on his publication record, in fact, Dr. Lee tended to pursue the research that most interested him at a given time, working to the utmost with the equipment and facilities available to him. This last comment should not be taken as celebratory, contributing to the construction of a heroic figure but, rather, as an observation on Lee's managerial skills in his capacity as the chief administrator of his program. Rather than mastering a limited set of practices beginning in 1961, perhaps an appealing alternative under the circumstances, he took the opposite approach, pushing to develop his program as fully and as rapidly as possible, consistently mobilizing the ambitious vocabulary of a cardiac surgery community.

In this respect, Dr. Lee's efforts at building international links should be seen not simply as part of the process of technical learning nor strictly as an effort to place himself within a network of suppliers. Rather, the act of network building represents a form of authentication, accommodating the risks associated with heart surgery by providing reassurance in the form of external validation through international partners. If it would be some time before South Korean patients would seek out the hospital facility on their own, the quickest way to provide them with certainty lay not only in a record of providing service and successful surgeries but also in the visibility of these external partnerships. This trend is true for much of South Korean higher education as well, in which the majority of faculty members hold terminal degrees from American or European universities; the practice holds for medicine as well, where visiting clinical fellowships testify to a surgeon's expertise.

In Dr. Lee's case, the nine-month clinical rotation in Europe, spanning September 1965 to June of the next year, added luster to his two years in Minneapolis (from 1957 to 1959), granting him a cumulative experience that would serve his career well. This does not mean that his material circumstances in Seoul changed dramatically; in fact, quite the contrary. A letter of July 1967 to Dr. Lillehei offers a stance similar to the one taken prior to the Sweden venture, noting that "things are really slow-moving for my work here," referring to a lack of "oxygenator lines and parts."[111] However, the tone is now a committed one, recognizing that "with basic equipment at hand I could make progress in open heart surgery field."[112] That is, the vocabulary has changed considerably from the despair of August 1965, with the critical difference lying in the emerging language of development and international exchange, a set of phrases that Dr. Lee was now mastering to a high degree and was quick to mobilize.

In this same letter, in fact, Dr. Lee closes his remarks with a boost of confidence, stating that "as soon as I get my expendable supplies I am looking forward to go in open heart cases more vigorously."[113] Specifically, the emphasis here rests on equipment to be provided by SIDA, a gas monitor and electrodyne cardiac monitor, with both designed for use in surgery. The trip to Sweden had brought a significant change to his perspective on surgery, and he no longer cited personal shortcomings as a source of delays to the program. Instead, the problem is framed almost entirely in terms of bureaucracy, in particular, an economy of technical parts, with these tools permitting access to better forms of care. The shift here is a subtle one, as Dr. Lee still placed a high degree of trust in his equipment, but this questions the logic behind its lack of availability, even as he accepted his position in a country where these objects were "very difficult or almost impossible to be procured."[114]

In short, Dr. Lee had become a very different type of surgeon by the second half of 1966, and while we should not make too much of his personal transformation, the key distinction here lies in his attitude, a renewed willingness to mobilize the South Korean program as something valid, a position very different from the stance he took as late as mid-1965. With this approach, Dr. Lee was prepared, moreover, as SNU hospital made plans to formally declare the opening of its thoracic surgery program in 1968, feeling that it had successfully passed out of its initial developmental stages. In a period of approximately a decade, from 1958 to 1968, the hospital had gone from a location with a limited availability of beds, relying almost exclusively on outpatient visits, to a biomedical research site, where patients formed a critical part of an ambitious clinical program. The relationships that SNU surgeons had formed with international partners provided further opportunities for skill acquisition and, more important, testified to the reliability and credibility of the site, representing a form of external validation.

This credibility also took the form of a revamped surgical practice by late in the decade, with the clinical program representing an emerging hybrid, constituting a blend of South Korean practice combined with the new elements borrowed from several international partners, primary among them the Americans and the Scandinavians. The establishment of clinical rounds and new professional categories in the late 1950s at SNU resulted in a much higher degree of specialization a decade later, with residents and interns available to serve alongside the surgeon. Whereas surgeons had generally attempted heart procedures with at most two physicians in 1960, the same space would be much more crowded by 1968, with attending specialists assuming the duty of monitoring respiration and other relevant tasks.[115] In effect, the use of the operating theater in this fashion represented a compromise, with a hierarchical culture still very much present as Korean surgeons translated what they had learned into new working habits.

Within the next decade, Dr. Lee and SNU Hospital built on these trends within the Asian region, and Lee took on new responsibilities both at the national level and in regional Asian organizations in his capacity as a heart surgeon. Again, this expanded role is not significant by itself but rather for what it says about the ambitions of the heart surgery community to participate in these forms of transnational activity. Only by reaching out to its partners could the SNU team achieve the successful replication of the surgical procedure, a stark contrast to the "black box" model of technology transfer, in which a fixed object relocates from one point to another. Moreover, the procedure required a radical shift in attitudes and approach toward human anatomy, as the human body became an object of research, something from which new knowledge could be gained.

If the focus on the body brought with it a new form of surgical culture, it would also need to accommodate the state's schemes for exploring the growth of health care as an option. Although the Park Chung Hee state would make its first overtures in this direction in 1963, the degree to which substantive change took place remains open to question, as most scholars locate the provision of health insurance late in the following decade, in 1977. Certainly the image of the South Korean hospital was improving, and both the size of the medical community and the activities of its health care professionals were undergoing corresponding changes.

The Medical/Clinical and Promoting Social Change: Practices and Attitudes?

If the human body had become an object of biomedical research in South Korea by the late 1960s, this statement does not mean that the act of performing surgery was by any means a common one nor that it was widely accepted. For this to happen, the hospital had to embrace a very different approach toward the provision of health care, and this transition came only with the provision of insurance coverage and the period of economic growth corresponding to the mid- to late 1980s. For Lee Young-Gyun, as with many other surgeons, this meant that along with the adoption of a new style of medical pedagogy came a much more aggressive attitude with respect to the recruitment of clients who could pay for their treatment, something not generally encouraged at large public hospitals. As he continued to integrate the lessons of both Minneapolis and Upsalla into his practice, therefore, Dr. Lee contemplated a future when he could extend his interests beyond SNU hospital, possibly even beginning his own practice.

In the decade immediately following the start of the thoracic surgery program, from 1968 to 1981, Dr. Lee spent the majority of his time at SNU in a senior role, continuing to develop his practice and skills. In the mid-1970s, he had the opportunity to pursue an additional refresher course of study, spending several months at the end of 1976—October through December—in the United States, this time based at the Mayo Clinic and in Texas. Along with these activities, he assumed an increasing number of honorary and bureaucratic titles, becoming in the process one of the most prominent cardiac physicians in South Korea and indeed in the northeast Asian region by the late 1970s. His letters to Dr. Lillehei from this period indicate a deepening satisfaction with his professional career and personal circumstances, and he did not leave the hospital for the pursuit of commercial gain per se, although he continued to look for additional means of developing his research interests.

For Dr. Lee, this pursuit meant an alternative that took the form of a new institute devoted exclusively to the heart, a space where he could exercise a high degree of control over his surroundings. Opening in late 1982, the Sejong Heart Institute, with financial backing provided by the Hyewon Medical Foundation, became one of the first sites in South Korea to offer specialized clinical training to heart surgeons exclusively, a focus permitting a high degree of specialization. Although the clinical setting at SNU in the late 1960s had permitted a handful of cases on an annual basis, the new site, with the latest equipment and a full support team to address the problems of control, began to handle cases in the hundreds from its second year of operation. Moreover, with an affiliation at SNU, Sejong served as an elite research setting, continuing the process of bringing South Korean cardiovascular care up to a level where patients would feel comfortable with the idea of having the surgery in Seoul.

This last remark highlights the reality that for much of the preceding period South Koreans requiring serious surgery, especially heart surgery, continued to travel abroad if they could afford it, despite improvements to Korean care. Indeed, the wife of South Korean president Chun Doo Hwan was affiliated with a charitable foundation assembled precisely for this purpose in the early 1980s, and she often brought young patients to accompany her when she traveled.[116] As it turned out, this foundation allowed for personal gain on the part of its senior members, with the foundation funding research, while also allowing sufficient space for financial manipulation of its funds. Although these remarks should not cast doubt on the valuable work performed at the Sejong Heart Institute, they do emphasize that the transition to a commercially viable South Korean surgical culture was one marked by a lengthy period of familiarization. To return to the point at which this chapter began, the Minnesota Project even went so far as to offer a small payment to the families of patients as a form of incentive in the early 1960s to induce this kind of change in behavior.

In closing this chapter, this curious incident from 1962 provides a fascinating coda to this period of intersecting medical and cultural change. In the last years of the Minnesota Project (in 1960 through 1962), senior American advisors implemented an incentive scheme designed to encourage their Korean counterparts to engage more deeply with the new clinical culture. Specifically, Korean doctors were given the sum of 500 won (the equivalent of about US$8) to persuade the families of their Korean patients to donate the body of a loved one for autopsy and further research. This unusual exchange reinforces the relative lack of clinical culture at SNUH at this time; indeed, nationwide numbers provided by ministerial records tend to support this claim. There remains much more to say about this practice from the standpoint of medical anthropology, of course, but for now, the point stands that the space of the Korean hospital changed only at an incremental pace, and that the changes did not necessarily translate immediately to the surrounding culture. South Korea began to change its attitudes about the body and health only with the start of large-scale public health campaigns coinciding with the arrival of a new government after 1961.

II Meet the State

4 Family Planning and Nation Building in South Korea, 1961 through the mid-1970s

Greeting the State (1966)? Distributing "New" Forms of Public Health

In 1966, the South Korean government began to sponsor mobile transportation as part of its national family planning (FP) effort, sending a series of vans to outlying areas to provide greater access to new birth control technologies and related services.[1] With echoes of previous efforts conducted first during the period of Japanese colonialism and later by a small subset of private interests under President Syngman Rhee (1948–1960), this "new" FP mobilization had officially begun two years earlier in 1964, with the distribution of the Lippes loop marking its inception.[2] Although the loop represented a new form of technology that the Population Council, the international organization founded by John D. Rockefeller III (1906–1978) in 1952, was eager to promote, the conjoined problems of its distribution and a need for accompanying reproductive education remained major issues, particularly in developing countries with a significant rural population.[3] In early accounts provided by observers during the South Korean mobile transportation campaign, these issues tend not to emerge explicitly, however, and published accounts often presented an idealized procession of eager, willing recipients:

> About 30 women are standing under the overhanging eaves of the township office building. They have finished filling out the record forms and are waiting patiently for the FP mobile clinic to open for business. They have signed up for loops [Lippes loop]. One woman leans against the building. She has walked

seven miles since daybreak. Two men are standing some distance from the women. They have signed up for vasectomies.[4]

It might not come as a surprise that this account originates with an American observer, Paul Hartman (1911–1968), who spent much of his time based in South Korea, working first for USAID (U.S. Agency for International Development) and subsequently for the Population Council, primarily in the field of health education.[5] As on-the-ground coordinator for the Population Council's South Korea program, Hartman had a great deal invested in the success of this effort, both personally and professionally.[6] This is not to discount his observations but rather to call attention to the smooth narrative with which he characterizes interactions among the van, the reproductive technologies to be delivered, and members of its target demographic, in this case, a small group of Korean villagers. In particular, Hartman emphasizes the enthusiasm of these participants, citing the great distance traveled by one woman while also noting the presence of two males who have volunteered to undergo a vasectomy, with males also constituting a key demographic as a major component of the FP mobilization.

The presence of these vans underscores a basic paradox underlying the South Korean effort: an attempt to accelerate the distribution of birth control technologies in a new nation essentially lacking a viable public health network outside of its major cities and also lacking a consistent and reliable means of delivery for reproductive education via mass communications. Like birth control itself, mobile vans had made an appearance on at least one previous occasion, with the American-Korean Foundation (AKF) employing a similar strategy during its relief efforts in the aftermath of the Korean War.[7] The FP campaigns, while not strictly "new" in the forms of technology offered, would ultimately be characterized as "successful" precisely because of their ability to consolidate resources and strategies borrowed from previous campaigns—often to much better effect—bringing pedagogy and technology together for large sections of the country over the course of the program's first decade of operations. As this chapter argues, the FP campaigns were critical not only for the degree and extent of bodily intervention achieved by the program and its representatives but also for their strategic use of various media, employing mass communications at the level of technology (television, radio, print) and even on the ground, placing FP representatives and agents directly into rural villages through the use of Mother's Clubs.

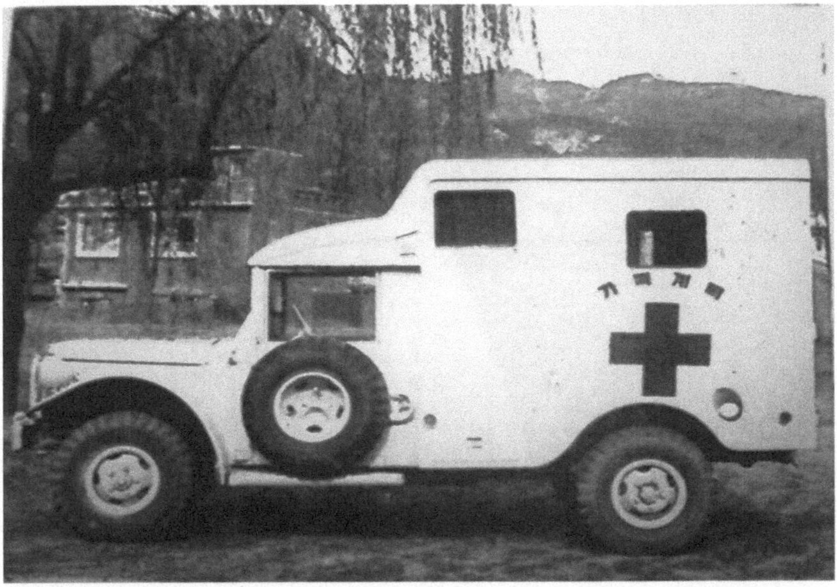

U.S. Army van, used in mobile services for family planning (FP) beginning in 1966. The text (above the Red Cross symbol) indicates "Family Planning." The program would also deploy a fleet of Volkswagens as part of its mobile transport effort to penetrate rural areas throughout South Korea, dramatically expanding the scope of health care.

Source: Mobile Service 1966, Courtesy of Rockefeller Archive Center.

To return to a point raised at the close of the preceding chapter, a general discomfort with the autopsy was extremely common in much of South Korea through at least the early to mid-1960s, corresponding to roughly the same time period as these mobilization efforts on behalf of FP. This suggests a conspicuous lack of fit between the program's aims and the existing practice of the population; in fact, the various parties involved—including representatives of Planned Parenthood Federation of Korea (PPFK) (Taehan Kajok Kyehoek Hyŏphoe), medical professionals, and a wide range of international partners—actively sought to enforce dramatic changes in the attitudes and behavior of South Koreans through the mechanism of public health, focusing specifically on mobilizing new reproductive and population policies. In brief, it was the FP campaigns, more than anything else, that brought a heightened awareness of public health concerns to South Korean villages and, more important, first introduced dramatic changes in attitudes toward the body, reproductive health, and any number of related forms of medical intervention.

These changes did not come easily, though, and much of the work of this chapter involves documenting the complex negotiations taking place among the state, the FP program, and citizens at a time of rapid social ferment. Although the earliest developments associated with the build-up and mobilization of the campaign—the distribution of the Lippes loop (1964), the use of mobile transportation (1966), followed by a change in emphasis to the birth control pill (1968)—coincided with the gradual strengthening of Park Chung Hee's hold over the ROK state apparatus, the FP campaigns ultimately had a much longer lifespan and impact as measured over the long term. By the early to mid-1970s, the activities of the *saemaŭl undong*, or the New Village movement, included FP as a major component situated within a broader campaign of rural revitalization, meaning that FP was actively promoted by the ROK state through at least the early to mid-1980s. Assuming a variety of different forms over its lifespan, family planning constituted a major part of South Korean social and cultural practice for more than two and a half decades (from 1964 through the mid-1980s), effectively bringing the ROK state and its emerging public health network directly into the domestic sphere; more specifically, the family and married life.

This campaign, or more properly series of campaigns, not only transformed domestic life but also brought with it a major overhaul of the governing bureaucracy, along with the South Korean academy, incorporating new models and approaches drawing from a wide variety of academic disciplines, especially the social sciences. More specifically, demography, a subject of intense interest to foreign visitors like Dr. Irene Taeuber as early as the late 1940s, began to take on a greater significance with the return of the first Korean graduate students to receive doctoral degrees in the field, now prepared to take up academic posts.[8] In practice, this meant that the type of statistical models and surveys needed for population estimates, as well as the underlying types of social science used to conduct interviews throughout the FP campaigns, was itself very much a development in process, a hybrid of earlier practices compiled during the colonial period, combined with the new perspectives emerging from leading demographic centers, including frequent exchange with the University of Michigan's Population Studies Center (PSC), Princeton University's Office of Population Research (OPR), and the University of North Carolina's Carolina Population Center (CPC), among others.[9]

In public health, similarly, the effort would be led by an emerging set of South Korean elites, many of whom possessed prior Japanese higher education and subsequent periods of American training, if not always taking a second terminal degree. Dr. Kwon E Hyock (1923–) of Seoul National University, holding a master's degree from the University of Minnesota via his participation in the Minnesota Project (1956), assumed leadership of a two-year pilot study conducted within the city limits of Seoul proper, labeled the Seongdong-gu (Sŏngdong-gu) Action Plan (1964–1966), a project that encompassed a large section of southeastern Seoul adjoining the northern banks of the Han River.[10] Concerned with substandard housing and living conditions in a densely populated urban area, Dr. Kwon's task was to disseminate basic information about reproductive health and to explain options available to women. More important, this pilot study went on to form a major portion of the practice and ideas shaping the subsequent national FP campaign.

At the same time, the Seongdong-gu study also led to recognition that the distribution of new technologies and the FP message was not a simple matter, even with the dense concentration of urban residents in sites like Seoul and a cluster of other major cities. As much of South Korea remained tied to the village and agrarian life, these residents did not necessarily "meet" the state on any regular basis, with the possible exception of routinized transactions such as taxation and military conscription. In this respect, the FP mobilization comprised not just a population or quantitative scheme but also a means of conveying new infrastructure (public health, reproductive education), with the package including a strong dose of nation building, fueling a sense of nascent nationalism that had been interrupted by the intervention of the Korean War. The publicity materials and posters associated with the campaign came to rely heavily on visual appeals to the nation, particularly the social and economic welfare of the collective as imagined through the family unit.

In some cases, as with the earliest posters provided by PPFK, this nationalist appeal would be much more implicit, embedded within an implied collective "we," one emphasizing the long-term benefits of the FP program as measured primarily by the health and welfare of South Korean children. For example, one of the first efforts to depict the face of the national campaign, circulated widely in 1965, depicts a female FP representative pointing to a Lippes loop (upper left), with two young children, a boy and a girl, an ideal pair in terms of both number and gender—although these concerns were not made explicit until much later—looking on in appreciation.[11] The accompanying text offers viewers encouragement to "have the appropriate number of children and raise them well!" (in Korean: *"Almatke naasŏ hullyunghage kirŭja!"*), a message

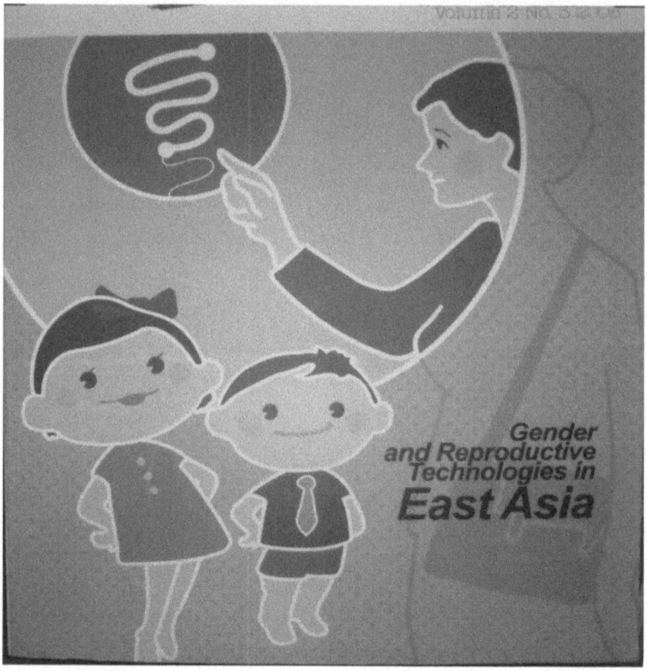

This 1965 poster introduced Family Planning to South Korea in the form of an FP representative explaining the Lippes loop and its proper use to two young children. The gender balance here explicitly challenges the traditional preference for sons, and the number of children, two, reinforces the goal of smaller families. English text not featured in the original poster.

SOURCE: PPFK.

placing an optimistic face on the future.[12] Although most of the FP program's major features are mobilized here—the technology, a female FP representative, and the desired end—members of the target demographic, young women in their reproductive years (defined by PPFK as in the age range of twenty to forty-four), are present only by implication, presumably included as members of the viewing audience.

Along with related materials supplied by PPFK, including posters and slogans, this particular image serves as a valuable introduction to the unique set of tensions embodied by the program, a national campaign situated within the interests of a set of competing actors, including South Korea and its international partners. The vast majority of the funding for the South Korean FP campaigns derived from abroad, including most prominently the Population

Council (Rockefeller) and SIDA (Sweden International Development Authority), with the latter group taking on an even greater role following the introduction of the birth control pill in 1968.[13] Under these circumstances, many of the campaign's posters were designed in conjunction with these outside actors, composed first with an international audience in mind and then translated to meet the needs of a local audience.[14] The priority of meeting national goals and targets frequently came into conflict with the abstract ideals of an international effort; these moments of tension, especially in terms of material practice, will serve to highlight the competing motivations and ambitions of the PPFK, the South Korean government, and those of its external partners.

Mobilizing a "New" FP Campaign (1961–1963)

Models and Precedents

It is precisely this brand of tension, introduced by the numerous differences between a set of enthusiastic, international actors and their ambitious local counterparts, that makes this period fascinating, with the early 1960s witnessing the start-up of comparable FP programs throughout much of East and Southeast Asia. Matthew Connelly, a historian at Columbia University, has even gone so far as to place this regional story within a much larger, international history of postwar family planning in his recent work *Fatal Misconception* (2007), attempting to narrate the Asian story as one of overzealous Cold War social science.[15] Although Connelly's account remains a valuable contribution, it relies almost exclusively on the perspective of the Population Council and its American partners, looking at material practice only briefly and relying on a number of top-down assumptions. Similarly, accounts that prioritize the individual nation and its corresponding FP story tend to ignore the transnational circulation of ideas and medical practices among new nations, a highly relevant point for South Korea specifically, where the influence of Japan—both in terms of colonial practice, and now in terms of providing expertise through visiting consultants and scholars—and Taiwan would be marked.[16]

In fact, Taiwan's pilot project at Taichung (1963), established and conducted with the assistance of Dr. Ronald Freedman (1917–2007) of the University of Michigan, became widely known as the first and best model for international FP, with both American and Taiwanese scholars continuing to generate publications on this basis for the better part of the next decade.[17] Along with Dr. John Y. Takeshita (1926–) and a rotating series of graduate assistants from Michigan, Dr. Freedman built his career as a demographer around the Taiwan program, which, like the South Korean case, intersected heavily with existing policy initiatives, including those previously promoted by both the KMT and the Japanese.[18] The extent to which this overlap was known to the Michigan team members in Taiwan remains speculative, but in the South Korean case there could be no mistaking the presence of these earlier forms of practice, both in terms of the technologies and local perceptions of these forms of intervention.[19] The challenge in 1961, therefore, lay with providing a convincing rationale behind a national campaign, one that could successfully render the program effectively as "new" in terms of the reception of its aims and practice.

Although official announcement of the FP effort would not come until 1964, when the program would go national in scale, the origins of a nascent program nearly coincided with the arrival of a new government, resulting in the formation of the PPFK (Planned Parenthood Federation of Korea) in April 1961.[20] While there had been similar efforts conducted at the grassroots level throughout the second half of the 1950s, the government of Syngman Rhee had never offered its full endorsement, possibly because of religious objections, along with the simultaneous burden of conducting extensive reconstruction efforts.[21] Affiliation with the international organization of the same name came later that year (June 1961), effectively linking the local group with its international partners, establishing the basis for the development of a large-scale effort.[22] The intervening years (1961–1963) prior to the scaling up of the program were devoted to making contact with regional and international partners, including site visits to Taichung to evaluate the comparable program in Taiwan and providing preparatory training to local health care professionals, the corps of doctors, nurses, and trainees who performed much of the actual work underlying the effort.

This brief account should not suggest, however, that the creation of a national program was a simple matter; recall from the previous chapter that many South Koreans were neither aware of, nor were they necessarily willing to make use of, newer forms of health care available to them through biomedicine. In effect, the FP effort united these two related strands: first, requiring a vast overhaul of health infrastructure—including health care facilities and the training of new professionals—and second, finding an effective means to disseminate information about the provision and availability of these services. Moreover, there were not enough trained doctors and nurses to mobilize a national campaign; when the widespread distribution of technologies began after 1964, the campaign turned frequently to its trainees and related categories of actors to perform many of the critical functions, such as the insertion of the Lippes loop.[23] This observation provides additional context to the mobile van image with which this chapter opened, bringing the technologies to rural areas but not without experiencing any number of related complications.

Even prior to the problem of accepting the technology as an issue, the very nature of an aggressive social science itself raised serious questions about whether such an ambitious campaign was worth attempting. The three-year period (1961–1964) leading up to the national mobilization reflects the care with which the effort came into being, with the establishment of a bureaucracy requiring the setup of individual branches at the city, provincial, and county levels.[24] Similarly, visits to Taichung in 1963 provided access to a rich source of data from a comparable site: a neighboring nation with reliable sources of population data dating to the late nineteenth century, a lingering Japanese presence from recent history, and a KMT government eager to implement rapid change. For Taichung specifically, the initial setup treated the entire city as an experimental context, with several different zones established—differentiated principally by the degree of media coverage and the types of information provided—to test the effectiveness of contrasting levels of media saturation.[25]

Through its varied approach, Taichung offered a variety of options to South Korea, giving the ROK the opportunity to observe before actively undertaking its own program. The social science coming from American sources took a particularly aggressive stance in assuming that its target subjects *invariably wanted* to use at least some form of birth control if only these groups possessed awareness of its availability. The data collection tools documenting this phenomenon, known as the "KAP surveys" (for "Knowledge, Attitude, and Practice"), created explicit links among awareness, a set of existing beliefs, and the ability of the social scientist to transform these attitudes through education, resulting in the adoption of new forms of practice. Like the Taiwanese, the South Koreans adopted this type of research in the near future, but prior to 1964 a "national" campaign existed only on paper as a bureaucratic organization, first seeking a means to establish reliable communications links across the southern half of the peninsula.

This last remark suggests that there was already a baseline level of research activity; in fact, as noted earlier, there were numerous continuities with the public health efforts of the late 1950s. As early as December 1963, the *Yonsei Medical Journal* (3.1) would publish the initial results of the Koyang study, a survey of attitudes toward family planning undertaken in a rural area close to the Seoul metropolitan area.[26] With research commencing in September 1962, this effort, headed by Dr. Jae-Mo Yang (1920–) of Yonsei University, along with his two collaborators, Sook Bang and Man Gap Lee, was likely the first attempt to evaluate the target demographic of the forthcoming national campaign.[27] As Dr. Yang had already conducted previous health surveys in the second half of the previous decade, he was familiar with the infrastructural problems of the South Korean health system and the skepticism directed toward it by a good portion of the population.

Dr. Yang's study—which extended well into the decade and also led to a number of follow-up efforts, typically based around village communities—represented the starting point of what became a vast social science industry, with senior figures leading new projects and junior Korean scholars using their affiliations to earn overseas doctoral degrees. This pattern suited the South Korean context well, as it ensured their international partners that the distribution of funds and reproductive technologies were overseen by a set of reliable counterparts on the ground, operating according to the same basic set of assumptions, with new actors playing a prominent role on their return home. Along with Dr. Kwon's Seungdong-gu study, the Koyang research provided a dual strategy of access to South Korean domestic life, concentrating on both the rural (Koyang) and urban (Seungdong-gu), as the ROK government sought to assess its ability to penetrate the home and intervene in the reproductive lives of citizens. As Dr. Yang knew from his previous work, the problem was rarely as simple as conveying the technology to the user but was in fact a far more complex one of conveying an appropriate message to village residents, who did not necessarily possess any incentives to change their behavior.

Pursuing "Demographic Dividends": Family Planning and Economic Incentives (1962–1964)

Yonsei University and the Koyang Study (1962): From the Individual to Statistical Abstraction

In fact, this question of the individual was not a major issue, as the rhetoric and practice of the FP program was based almost entirely on a new conception of improving the economic fortunes of the country by establishing control over the population as a set of abstract calculations. Even as the language of public health and improved living conditions figured prominently in the literature of the nascent program, its major goals were defined in statistical terms: Achieving a certain quota of distribution was likely to yield well-defined results in terms of a reduced population, with this development producing better economic circumstances. In one of the preliminary reports issued in conjunction with the Koyang study, this goal was made explicit to an international audience, with an anonymous contributor from the Population Council noting that the ROK "aims at a large increase in [its] gross national product."[28] This aim was achieved by halving the population increase rate within a period of about two decades (by 1980), a modest claim in retrospect, as the program actually achieved its results much earlier than this.

Although these aims were constructed largely in mathematical terms, the target demographic was rendered in slightly more concrete terms, with a loose conception of modernization theory framing the approach taken by the participating social scientists, whether South Korean or visiting from abroad. Dr. Yang and the members of his team chose their site for its proximity to Seoul, with Koyang based approximately thirteen miles north of Seoul and featuring an existing site for the training of medical students affiliated with Yonsei/Severance Hospital. Moreover, the rural character of the site held particular appeal, with such areas often having a higher birth rate and generally lacking prior exposure to the new birth control technologies coming onto the market. In other words, this was precisely the type of population to offer an ideal test case of the proposition that an informed population would readily adopt the new measures and begin the desired FP style of practice on learning of its availability. In terms of its proximity and design, this type of village area offered the potential to suit the expectations of the emerging social science.

The force of two conjoined issues, a lack of awareness and education, provided a rationale for much of the program's motivation, which assumed eager and willing participants on the receipt of appropriate information. According to this methodology, these willing subjects should adopt family planning measures, rapidly increasing the pool of those practicing some form of "modern" birth control.[29] Collectively, this newly enrolled cohort would then produce a smaller and healthier group of children, resulting in education and health care savings for the state, thereby leaving additional funds to invest in the infrastructure necessary to promote industrial and economic growth. According to this design, incremental increases in the size of the population following the program's dictates later translated into significant gains for the state in terms of sources of revenue and future economic projections. These "demographic dividends," as the optimistic projections were characterized, informed the program's larger aims, even as they were not always made explicit in the encounter with the individual subject.

This encounter between state and citizen, whether taking place in the street, in the clinic, or at even closer quarters within the village and the home, proved to be incredibly problematic as the international proponents of family planning tended to adopt an implicit universalism, taking for granted the opportunity to establish face-to-face communication across a wide range of cultural contexts.[30] However, with South Korea representing only one case of the problem, this basic format envisioned a highly literate population with access to several different forms of media (print, radio, and television) and with a corresponding curiosity; in other words, a willingness to embrace change. As the Koyang study showed, the encounter with the village resident was a highly mediated one, shaped by previous encounters with health care and perhaps even with lingering memories of different governing regimes (Japan, USAMGIK). The distribution of birth control technologies, in other words, was not simply an issue of a technological object in isolation but rather an entire cultural package and the sets of values and aspirations associated with it.

When the Koyang study began in September 1962, this long-range perspective was lacking, and there remained a great deal of optimism concerning the possibility of interacting directly with villagers close to their home environment. Dr. Yang and his Yonsei team divided the community in terms of their experimental design, designating an experimental area and a control area so as to be able to compare results. Concerned with the question of interpersonal dynamics, they next selected from among a small group of graduate students—including Yonsei medical students and, in some cases, local midwives—before choosing two groups of ten males and ten females to interview exclusively villagers of the same gender. Essentially, the study was designed to keep intervention in village life to a minimum and to establish a baseline estimate, determining the extent to which the government's intention of starting a family planning program may have already penetrated this designated area outside of Seoul.[31]

After accounting for factors such as dropouts and slight differences between the two target populations, what the survey ultimately found was the value of interpersonal communication, a point of emphasis that became critical within the national program by 1968. Specifically, the first publication emerging from the project noted that "personal communication between friends, relatives and neighbors is the commonest means of acquiring knowledge," especially in areas lacking access to new forms of mass communication.[32] While this point was not an immediate cause for action, it did lead to two subsequent suggestions: namely, that any future program should focus on education aimed at small groups, precisely to take advantage of this close level of dialogue; and to target both males and females, enabling couples to share information at home and to make an informed decision together.[33] Though modest in its size and cost, the Koyang study proved highly influential in terms of the forthcoming national mobilization.

The Seongdong-gu Action Plan (1964–1966)

If the Koyang study provided the basis for much of the long-term strategy in terms of designing a new approach to disseminate information about the FP program, its counterpart, the Seongdong-gu study sponsored by Seoul National University, was equally significant: Here the urban residents of Seoul met the infrastructure of the state in the form of public health. In the case of Koyang, Yonsei had relatively little infrastructure to work with, creating its own temporary clinic as part of an outreach program, combining a blend of research and humanitarian motives. In the case of Seongdong-gu, the initial aims had much less to do with communication, focusing instead on broad themes of urban renewal, a coded vocabulary for slum removal and access to basic necessities such as clean water and reliable housing.[34] The rural problem of a high number of births—reaching an estimated six per woman during childbearing years as of 1960—remained a major theme, but here the emphasis was placed on reproductive pedagogy and improving relations between the state and potential client. How could the state provide adequate care and reproductive education as its cities continued to grow rapidly; more important, how might it persuade residents to make use of these facilities?

The Seongdong-gu section of Seoul encompassed a broad strip of the southeast, stretching from the traditional city center to reach the northern banks of the Han River. While the sections lying directly opposite, the southern banks of the Han River, came to represent some of the newest and wealthiest areas of Seoul within less than twenty-five years, the study's focus on the region at this time was motivated primarily by a rapidly growing population and the social problems typically associated with such urban spaces—sanitation, disease, and housing. Moreover, the proximity of the Seoul National University main campus, based at Taehan-ro, provided for ease of access, like the Koyang study, permitting medical students and public health experts ready availability to a site close to their home base. With the national campaign starting in 1964, Seongdong-gu experienced the added pressure of conducting its activities more or less on a simultaneous basis, that is, setting up a clinic on site at the same time that distribution of the loop technology was just getting underway.

As a result, this project arguably took on a greater visibility than its counterpart in Koyang, situated within city limits where local residents had access to its facilities and services, which was, after all, precisely the point of constructing such a site. The project could accommodate the need for adjustments midcourse, if necessary, but there would be no turning back once committed or reverting to earlier forms of practice. In its material presence, Seongdong-gu placed its emphasis on the creation of infrastructure for the delivery of health services, a major point that continued through at least the first decade of the FP program. Although citizens still did not possess confidence in biomedicine, sometimes opting not to use the state's new resources in the form of hospitals or health centers—as limited as these sites were in the early 1960s—the state assumed the initiative to meet its citizens.[35] Over the course of its lifetime, before it was gradually absorbed within the broader rhetoric and practice of the rural revitalization campaigns of the 1970s, FP aggressively played the role of a major state actor in terms of the construction and the mobilization of such resources.

Together with Koyang, Seongdong-gu redefined the relationship between doctor and client, as the target demographic for FP was no longer an individual "patient" but instead an "acceptor," one who consented to use of a (new) birth control technology or, in the case of males, voluntarily agreed to undergo a vasectomy.[36] This language embodied the new social science deriving from the University of Michigan/KAP surveys, in which the dominant assumption took the willing participation of subjects for granted, contingent on access to the latest information and an appropriate program of education. Although this model implied an artificial distinction between the "traditional" and the "modern," placing these categories within a much larger body of midcentury literature on modernization, this was not a self-conscious or reflective gesture but instead one embodying the confidence of the program. Individual "acceptors" figured as significant only as measured in bulk, as the entire program was gauged as a success based on a statistical approach that measured increases in the distribution of technological objects.

Tracking Intervention through Technology: The Lippes Loop and Defining a "Modern" Birth Control (1964–1968)

Although the focus of the national FP effort placed its emphasis on tracking the distribution of birth control technologies, not every object would count as valid, with the focus resting almost exclusively on new objects provided by international partner nations, with some provision for a limited number of objects of Korean manufacture. Although existing practices, including herbal remedies to prevent pregnancy and the practice of "spontaneous abortion," were frequently noted in the course of KAP surveys, these practices served only as a baseline, a means against which to measure the spread of the more desirable, "modern" forms of birth control.[37] The Lippes loop, the product of a great deal of research into the creation of an easily transportable form of IUD, thus became the single most important technology during the early stages of the FP program (from 1964 through 1968), with its distribution constituting the primary criterion for success. Beginning in 1964, PPFK carefully tracked the distribution of these devices, along with the corresponding number of "acceptors," using survey data to make frequent adjustments to the campaigns as more data became available.

The aim of promoting distribution of the loop brought with it a number of problems, however, some of which we have already anticipated in the mobile van scene that opened this chapter. Designed for rapid insertion into the female body, the loop represented the most recent attempt to provide a safe, inexpensive means of preventing pregnancy. In fact, a limited number of Korean and Taiwanese women had prior exposure to IUDs in the form of the Ota ring, a prewar device created by a Japanese doctor; references to the object appeared beginning in the mid-1960s, experiencing a renewal of attention with the introduction of newer technologies.[38] Despite its compact design, however, the loop required a high degree of familiarity with its use, and the insertion procedure was by no means as simple as its creators would claim.[39] In basic terms, distribution of the loop was going to require not only the skills of survey workers who would gauge the attitudes of Korean women but also those of a corresponding pool of doctors, nurses, and trainees who would be there to provide counsel and to perform the necessary insertion procedure safely and effectively.

The Loop and Reproductive Education: Choosing from a "Menu"

Before turning to the activities of this second group, the professional caregivers, it is worth noting that the loop did not necessarily represent the most common item marked for distribution when the Seongdong-gu plan began, lagging behind condoms as the preferred choice at a rate of almost two to one.[40] In 1964, the IUD was initially placed among a range of options—condoms, foam tablets, jelly, and the loop—with the aim of establishing a baseline survey of market preferences.[41] At this point, the loop possessed a formidable image, involving an uncomfortable insertion procedure and the possibility of long-term use, characterizing it with uncertainty. New visitors to sites associated with the project opted more frequently for the condom and other technologies associated with either a single or short-term use, even as the loop would come to represent a significant share of the items to be distributed. To revisit a point made earlier, abortion remained a constant, comprising the single largest share of the family planning techniques then available, and it was precisely against these trends that PPFK mobilized its new devices.[42]

Preference for the loop began to change only with the added role of education and counseling, allowing it to catch and pass the condom within a period of two to three years. More specifically, potential "acceptors" were not pressured to opt for insertion immediately and were instead issued a coupon that could be redeemed for a follow-up visit leading to the actual insertion procedure. The measure of introducing an intermediate stage thereby allowed the Seongdong-gu team to track the pool of those interested and to determine what percentage of this pool would return for a subsequent visit. Moreover, this gesture rendered the loop as something new and novel, not necessarily as intimidating, but as a valuable service to be redeemed through the exchange of a coupon. Not surprisingly, the Seongdong-gu study found that a switch to the loop tended to correspond to those areas of the city receiving the greatest media saturation (exposure to advertisements, mail) and follow-up information sessions held in group settings. It required time and familiarity, in other words, allowing the individual "acceptor" a sufficient interval in which to make a personal decision.

With the city borders of Seoul forming the boundaries of the study, the focus on one region of the city would gradually expand to include eight additional subcenters, along with the original site at Seongdong-gu, over a period of about two to three years (from 1964 to 1967).[43] This incremental expansion in coverage allowed for a thorough test of the available techniques—mass media, home visits, and group meetings—to gauge the program's ability to disseminate its message. Although this level of saturation did not prove practical on a nationwide basis for this period in the mid-1960s, it is safe to say that the majority of the urban residents were exposed to some form of FP, with direct mail and subsequent group meetings forming the core of the approach. In preparation for the anticipated increase in demand for the loop, PPFK began to train increasing numbers of its personnel about the insertion procedure and about what to anticipate in terms of likely questions and the side effects associated with its use.

The Loop Becomes a Problem (1964–1968)

The Lippes loop represented a major investment on the part of the Population Council and other interested parties, the latest in a series of technological improvements to intrauterine devices, which had a history going back to at least the first half of the twentieth century with the Grafenburg ring.[44] Although such devices were generally effective in preventing pregnancy, the physical problems associated with their insertion and long-term use continued to present numerous problems, and the Lippes loop proved no exception. In its large form, the Lippes loop was expected to remain in the body for long periods of time, with an expected expulsion rate of slightly more than 12 percent and another 15 percent of subjects requesting medical removal.[45] Under optimal conditions, about 25 percent of its users could expect to experience problems with the device to a degree requiring its removal, and this estimate *does not* include the related physical discomfort and symptoms associated with "normal" use. In effect, South Korean women in the early 1960s were among those subjects serving as part of an unofficial clinical trial for the device throughout the developing world, a test case to evaluate its effectiveness and safety.[46]

When South Korean women first began to "meet" the state through FP beginning in 1964, the loop stood at the center of this encounter, with advocates seeking to persuade as many women as possible to become "acceptors," affirming the statistical goals of the program. When a coupon "acceptor" returned to a health center or clinic for a follow-up consultation, only then was the insertion procedure undertaken, placing the loop within her body, where it would remain, ideally, for a lengthy period of time. The conditions under which this procedure was performed, however, varied widely according to the site; even with the additional training funded by the Population Council, the shortage of doctors and nurses meant that trainees or field workers quite often oversaw this kind of work.[47] In spite of its design, moreover, crafted to permit ease of use, the loop did not necessarily lend itself to ready manipulation, meaning that discomfort frequently occurred both during the procedure itself and in subsequent use, especially when the device was not properly situated or, to borrow from the language of the program, there was a failure to achieve "skillful insertion."[48]

In follow-up studies of IUD use, the Seongdong-gu group found that a cluster of factors—including bleeding, discomfort, and related complaints about the device—grouped under the broad rubric of "medical side effects"—came to constitute the single largest cluster of motivations contributing to the increasing termination rate for the device.[49] This problem threatened to become a practical, as well as a public relations, embarrassment, so much so that this same set of studies later stated that "minimizing the removal rate is the most important issue" in determining the long-term efficacy of the loop.[50] Although there was recognition that the skill of participating doctors and their enthusiasm in promoting the device could play a significant role, "acceptors" as subjects also began to receive some of the blame for problems, with their symptoms minimized in resulting accounts. In particular, younger women with a high level of education were singled out for "their sensitivity to the mildest side effects, and the weak physiological tolerance of the uterus to foreign material."[51]

Improving Training and Technology

Along with this issue, the related question of training also came into play, as those responsible for the insertion more often than not received a bare minimum of instruction prior to performing their first procedure. A Population Council memo devoted to this subject cites a "large number of individuals with special training . . . [as] essential to the development of a successful program of family planning."[52] Having made this claim, the memo goes on to explain circumstances on the ground, with a curriculum "well-conceived and flexible enough to allow the number of hours of instruction to be varied from 12 to 64 to fit the needs and available time of each group."[53] Taking into account the contingencies of the time, the language sounds highly pragmatic and translates into a reality where many loop insertions were performed by an individual who had simply attended a brief training course. Granted, many of these individuals had prior training as midwives or as registered nurses, and in some cases both, but this memo underscores the program's heavy reliance on local personnel, placing a high degree of trust in their abilities.

This last statement holds for the dissemination of the training information as well, as the entire program was contingent on its pedagogy reaching from the national level down to the local village, grouped according to a network scheme that radiated from a central source. For FP, this source was the National Public Health Training Institute (Seoul), with Four Provincial Training Centers assuming a portion of the burden.[54] Another memo differs from the previous one in describing some of the feedback mechanisms, adding criticism and evaluation following each training session. At the same time, the emphasis remains clearly on timeliness and efficiency, permitting FP workers only a one- or two-week exposure through one of the training centers. In contrast to those performing the loop insertion, these FP workers were likely to be doing basic counseling and distributing information, but they still held a critical role in conveying the message to the public, especially with respect to unfamiliar procedures and technologies still largely untested.

If there remained questions about the difficulty of getting sufficient numbers of trained personnel into the field, the new forms of technology were equally at issue, especially their manufacture and reliability. At least officially, international partners provided the local FP representatives, the PPFK, with samples in quantities large enough to meet demand. In turn, the plan projected that South Korean manufacturers would later assume responsibility for their domestic production, meaning that the program would incorporate a useful dimension of industrial and technical learning. The reality was quite different, as a memo reveals that South Koreans began producing the loop on an independent basis as early as 1964, presumably as a cost-saving measure to avoid paying licensing fees.[55] Initially, this approach did not present problems, as the production fell under the domain of a plastics engineer, Mr. Han Bo Yoon, who oversaw the process from 1964 to 1967.[56] As demand grew, the Ministry of Health had to seek assistance from USAID, as it lost control over the local process in 1967 and had to acknowledge to its American partners that there "is no loop quality control system within the ministry."[57]

This admission posed a problem not simply as a potential source of embarrassment between friendly nations but also in terms of negative perceptions it might create, especially during the trial stages of the program. A 1964 memo provides further context to the discussion in the preceding paragraphs, with the Ministry of Health taking the stance that the "loop was not patented and that Korea was free to make them if it could."[58] Following the start-up of production, Dr. Jae-Mo Yang and others expressed concerns that using loops of both imported and domestic manufacture might compromise the validity of the preliminary FP studies, especially if there were significant differences in the end product.[59] In raising this issue, they soon learned that the medical advisers assigned to the program preferred to recommend the American loops, although they failed to cite specific criteria. Without offering speculation here, it is clear that the question of the technology raised the issue of its reliability, its source of manufacture, and its ease of use. Any of these factors, in isolation, or in combination, could potentially affect the perceptions of an "acceptor," leading an individual to discontinue its use or simply to refuse the device.

This observation brings us to perhaps the most important issue of all, the procedure for insertion, assuming the availability of trained personnel and access to the technology, both of which points were by no means a certainty, as we have just seen. Unlike the idealized accounts mobilized by PPFK and the state, this encounter, whether taking place in a clinic in Seoul or outdoors in a rural area with assistance from a mobile van, would have been new and largely unfamiliar to the vast majority of South Korean women. A 1967 manual distributed to FP workers precisely for this purpose provides a detailed set of instructions, attempting to translate the task in the form of a menu that can be followed along in both English and Korean-language versions.[60] This strategy seeks to reduce any ambiguity or uncertainty, accompanying the text with a set of detailed visual images, illustrating the placement of the plastic loop within the uterus. It is worth noting that the document begins with a "Worker's Creed," a pledge in which the target audience consents to "the task of stimulating as many eligible couples as possible to limit the number or spacing of their children through sterilization or use of the most effective contraceptives available."[61]

This creed is particularly important because it reinforces the agenda underlying the preceding statement concerning the aim of achieving a set of target figures. Specifically, the worker is asked to commit to the statement that "I will persuade as many as possible of the wives to try the loop method first even though I am fully aware that some 25% of them will not be able to tolerate or retain this device following insertion."[62] Here we have a direct acknowledgment of the physical problems associated with use, and yet even this knowledge is followed by reassurance that "I will recommend the loop as first choice . . . [because] I have no way of determining who the unlucky acceptor might be."[63] In effect, the logic of the document stresses the 75 percent rate of acceptance by the majority of women, thereby minimizing the suffering of one-quarter of the target group, displacing any responsibility on the part of the FP worker. In the end, the testing of the technology is what matters, and the creed closes with, "This is my job; securing as many new acceptors as possible and making sure that they become regular and satisfied users."[64]

As for the account of the insertion procedure, it implies the presence of a stable environment—a doctor's office or a comparable clinic facility—and involves a brief gynecological inspection, followed by cleaning of the cervix and vagina and a series of measured steps to ensure that the insertion is performed properly. Although the document intends to provide reassurance with its careful pace, it offers at the same time a recognition that mistakes could occur at any number of points, leading to an improper insertion. On this point, the number of steps comprising a complete insertion procedure, from initial contact to visual confirmation of insertion, is thirteen: Seven steps precede the procedure, allowing for a lengthy period of familiarization, with the final six steps comprising the actual insertion.[65] To return once again to the opening vignette of this chapter, it is not difficult to contrast the idealized account offered here in training with the mundane realities of the mobile clinic, typically operating in an outdoor, rural setting under a hot sun. In practice, many of these steps were omitted, yielding to the impulse to service as many "acceptors" as possible in a short period of time.

A 1969 publication appearing under the auspices of the Yonsei research group tends to affirm the likelihood of these pressures affecting practice, as the article—ostensibly a look at some of the statistical problems to be addressed—offered a frank look at the material conditions typically associated with the act of giving birth.[66] In rural settings, the vast majority of South Korean women bore their children in the home, most commonly the residence of their mother-in-law, and very rarely in a hospital setting.[67] Rather than a doctor, a relative or friend was most typically the individual present to provide assistance, if there was anyone available at all. As for their surroundings, newborn Korean babies often came into the world on the floor, with perhaps a straw mat or the paper bag from a cement sack providing a minimum of cover. Finally, the umbilical cord was generally cut with unsterile scissors and sometimes a sickle, when possible. With these rudimentary conditions common for the act of giving birth late in the decade, even following nearly five to seven years of intense FP mobilization, the circumstances help us to imagine the type of encounter that FP workers or trainees faced on a regular basis, with only limited time at each rural site.

The recognition of a growing problem with the loop took place gradually within the two- to three-year (from 1964 to 1967) period following its introduction, meaning that the program underwent major changes by the late 1960s. As noted earlier, the loop had figured prominently within a "menu" scheme—sometimes referred to as a "cafeteria," permitting "acceptors" to select from a range of options—through which it had risen to achieve great popularity. By 1968, the loop retained this position, but other options now received equal, and sometimes even greater, publicity, with the birth control pill receiving the full weight of the FP program's sponsorship. Measured strictly in quantitative terms, the loop had achieved enormous success, with the ROK government and its partners distributing large quantities of the technology, tracking its use and associated problems, and also managing to follow those individuals who had dropped out of the program. In fact, this last group proved of great interest to social scientists and demographers, not only for evaluation purposes but also in terms of designing new programs to bring these subjects back within the boundaries of the FP campaign.[68]

The subsequent labeling of this special group as "rejectors," those who chose to discontinue use of the loop based on their physical and psychological responses to the device, underscores a major issue for the program. If there were not enough personnel to meet the demand for proper insertion of the loop, or even basic health consultations, there were certainly not sufficient staff members to address the issue of follow-up care. FP was strictly quantitative in basing its approach at the front end, the entire goal being enrollment of the individual within the program, meaning the distribution and placement of technologies. The start of mobile van campaigns in 1966, with the intent of meeting increasing demand in rural areas, further emphasizes this point, as the vans were motivated primarily by distribution: These personnel did not necessarily expect to meet the "acceptors" in subsequent visits to the same location, which might not take place for at least several weeks, in any case. By the late 1960s, the problem of dropouts called attention to this issue, both in the form of conducting further studies and in designing supplemental forms of follow-up care.

The Male Role within Family Planning (1964–1968)?

The cluster of key issues associated with use of the loop—the need for careful insertion, follow-up care, and a number of personnel required to track those who opted out—were similar to those with respect to male reproduction, also a major part of FP but generally one receiving much less attention in the literature.[69] In fact, South Korean males represented a significant part of the target demographic from the program's inception, incorporated within the decision-making process for the family unit and instructed to begin using condoms on a more regular basis. Although the vasectomy ultimately proved a far more complicated means of addressing the problem, it is nonetheless remarkable that a significant number of individuals consented to the procedure, typically after they had achieved a family size that they deemed to be sufficiently large. In fact, the Seondong-gu Action Plan later included at least one case study of males adopting the vasectomy in the Seoul region late in the decade (July 1969), offering a fascinating portrait of the program's efforts to provide sufficient incentives for such a procedure.[70] We will look at both of these approaches, the condom and the vasectomy, in turn.

The Condom (1964–early 1968)

For much of this same period during which the Lippes loop was popular for women, condoms were distributed regularly as an option within the FP menu, and here the issue appears to have been primarily one of locating a reliable supply, an issue that we have already seen with the loop. Local firms sought to gain entry into the market as early as 1965, particularly the Dongkuk Condom Factory, leading to a complex series of negotiations between Population Council representatives based in New York and their counterparts around the world. In brief, the Population Council was pleased to locate a domestic partner but had serious questions about the reliability of Korean manufacturers. In the short term, the firm had to offer evidence of its products and their reliability, even obtaining a translation of their (Japanese) certificate of quality.[71] The Population Council also requested that additional testing be contracted out, a task to be performed in either England or the United States.[72] Even with these reservations, though, the Council still hoped to do business with the Korean firm, encouraging that Dongkuk begin to receive "some of [the] business from India, Pakistan, and Turkey."[73]

This last remark touches on the sensitivity of the product as critical to the perceptions of its end users. That is, Population Council representatives were concerned not only with reliability but also with how an object of domestic manufacture would be regarded by local users, to whom a condom manufactured abroad might easily appear to be a superior item. Shipping Dongkuk products abroad encouraged the firm in its business while allowing the Council to continue its work in South Korea unimpeded. This same issue emerged three years later, in 1968, as SIDA (Sweden International Development Cooperation Agency) began to first get heavily involved with the distribution of the birth control pill, in addition to condoms. A Swedish government representative, Stig Ljunggren, clarified his position with the Population Council, noting a good impression of Dongkuk, "an ambitious firm [that] . . . sooner or later . . . might come in business."[74] The problem lay once again with the condoms: "I am, however, not interested, in buying their machineries, but their condoms, so I have to keep to the quality of these ones."[75]

Ljunggren's remarks capture the tension surrounding a renewal of emphasis on the condom in the late 1960s, which would hold serious implications for the success or failure of the program. At least officially, the issue was not about commerce—that is, capturing a potential new market for condoms—but about ensuring the long-term viability of the FP program. As he put it later in the same document, Ljunggren observed that "I am sure I am right, when I say that quality is more important than price. A bad quality can spoil a whole programme."[76] Interestingly, he concluded in almost exactly the same fashion as the Population Council had previously in 1965, with a vague promise to purchase Dongkuk products in the future, offering them "as a gift from the Swedish Government to a developing country," the clear implication being a country other than South Korea.[77] Nearly four years into the FP program, the emergence of tensions like this indicated that a critical shift was taking place, with new international partners like Sweden joining the effort and with a growing awareness that the program was not functioning as effectively as it might.

At the same, it is critical to note here that the issue of South Korean males and their patterns of behavior regarding reproductive choices rarely emerged in conjunction with condom use, as the FP program assumed that greater familiarity would be sufficient to produce regular use. With the vasectomy, however, the acceptor/user would figure prominently in any conversation, as this was clearly a decision with more serious and lasting consequences. What types of incentives might appeal to Korean males, persuading them to undergo the procedure? Moreover, how might such a procedure be mobilized as a complement to existing FP initiatives?

Vasectomy: The Surgical Option (namsŏng purim susul)

As we briefly met two of these volunteers in this chapter's opening scene, it is useful to return to the scene and ask what type of individual was likely to opt for a vasectomy under these circumstances. Not surprisingly, the majority of those in this pool made the decision primarily on an economic basis, with their family size already placing a strain on their ability to provide and having heard about the procedure through either a friend, a family member, or a recommendation from a program representative. Roughly two-thirds of those interviewed were more than forty years old, with an average age of forty-two.[78] Building on this statistical portrait, the majority of these men had married in their early to mid-twenties, and by the time of the interview they had a family with an average size of four children, including on average of slightly more than two sons.[79] In a sense, these men had already achieved what they had hoped for and now sought a means of control, thereby limiting the number of their offspring.

Moreover, within the first decade of the FP program, there were significant numbers of these Korean men, the vast majority of them consenting to the procedure on a voluntary basis. In a 1971 assessment of the first decade of field operations, Dr. Jae-Mo Yang noted the quantitative success of the effort, which had set an annual quota aiming for 20,000 subjects for vasectomy beginning in the early 1960s.[80] Although these figures proved too ambitious for the early years, subsequent gains meant that the cumulative total approached nearly 200,000 subjects, despite the initial lag period.[81] These figures were achieved under difficult conditions, with a conspicuous shortage of doctors and trained personnel, meaning that our two volunteers at a mobile clinic site were not at all unusual but, rather, fairly representative of the conditions for such a procedure. Like the loop, the invasive character of the vasectomy procedure was minimized in the program's publicity materials, with many individuals returning to work within two to three days of surgery.

What made this development possible was a combination of factors, including the careful use of imagery, new forms of social mobility becoming available to the Korean male, and normalization of the surgical procedure. Although posters for voluntary sterilization were not as prevalent as those for female birth control, they relied on a similar set of carefully crafted images, with a heavy reliance on visual materials that could be easily understood. In a famous example, a watermelon is displayed in its two forms, containing seeds on the left, and with its seeds removed, on the right.[82]

The accompanying text is nearly rendered superfluous by the visual display, which establishes an analogy between the male reproductive organs and the seeds contained within the watermelon. While it is much more difficult to reconstruct the context or reception of this imagery—precisely how and why South Korean males might have found this type of material persuasive—what remains is the group portrait taken from this time, with economic motives dominating and with a significant proportion of these men coming from new types of white-collar jobs, frequently working as clerks and lower-level staff members.[83]

This basic portrait tends to hold true for many of the associated clinical studies conducted over the course of the second half of the 1960s, particularly those headed by Dr. Hui-Young Lee of the Department of Urology at Seoul National University Hospital.[84] Along with several colleagues, Dr. Lee published a number of clinical studies of the psychological and physical effects of vasectomy from a postsurgery standpoint, differentiating primarily between groups of private and subsidized patients.[85] This critical distinction underscores the role of the state and FP in promoting the procedure, as a significant proportion of male "acceptors" derived from this second group, comprising an estimated two-thirds of the total group. The rise in the acceptance rate, in other words, was made possible through a system in which subjects received their treatment essentially for free, with the surgery and follow-up covered by funds provided by government programs.

Although the eugenic implications of this practice remain clear within the broad aims of the program, this point was rarely made explicit, with the exception of occasional remarks, such as a telling observation in a PPFK official history that "vasectomy, which has been practiced on low income people since the beginning year of the program, will be continued."[86] This emphasis on extending financial aid to reach all segments of society embraced other methods of birth control as well, with the free distribution of reproductive technologies. For vasectomy specifically, the logic was to create a stable pool of "permanent sterilization," targeting approximately 3 percent of the population in their reproductive years, with the emphasis primarily on males.[87] In terms of the distinction between private patients and those receiving subsidies, the latter group also began to receive a small sum as compensation for recovery time and income lost from work, a practice that started in 1966.[88]

The logic behind this financial gesture was to provide an additional form of incentive, with FP citing a figure of approximately US$2.91 provided on average, a sum designated as equivalent to the wages lost due to the side effects of the surgery.[89] At the same time, this strategy also indicates the underlying tension associated with FP, with vasectomy specifically beginning to generate a negative image among Korean men. Despite favorable quantitative measures, the program begin to shift its emphasis in 1966 in conjunction with the data sets emerging from the nation's first Five Year Plan (from 1962 to 1966), seeking new means of spreading the message and increasing the receptivity of target populations. As noted, mobile transportation formed one critical part of this revised approach, reaching rural areas on a periodic basis, typically once every one to two months. The vans provided distribution of IUD technology and health consulting through participating trainees, with on-the-spot vasectomy consultation included as one of the services available.[90]

FP maintained its core focus on female reproduction, a point receiving greater emphasis with the shift to oral contraceptives in the late 1960s. For its part, vasectomy continued to be promoted as a complementary form of male participation, with new forms of incentives provided in terms of housing policies for new apartments and early release from home reserve training (*yebigun*) by the early 1970s.[91] Of these two policies, the latter measure continues to linger in the memory of many South Korean males, as FP counseling and lectures devoted to the vasectomy specifically formed an essential part of the process of decommissioning, preparing young soldiers prior to their return to the home and civilian life.[92] This type of pedagogy continued until at least the mid- to late 1980s, meaning that the majority of South Korean men were exposed to the state's message for a period lasting more than a decade. While never completely successful, the vasectomy campaigns underscore the extent to which Korean males had to remain open to the possibility of bodily intervention, even while remaining suspicious of its side effects.

To summarize the frenzied activity of these early years from 1964 to 1968, the FP program had started as a top-down effort in 1964, with the two pilot studies conducted by Dr. Yang Jae-Mo of Yonsei and Dr. Kwon E-Hyock of Seoul National providing reassurance to international partners and targeting rural and urban areas, respectively. The ongoing problem of loop rejection (1964–1968), tied to both production issues and the significant discomfort associated with the technology, finally forced change by 1968, both in terms of the primary objects of focus and the approach to be taken toward distribution and pedagogy. With assistance from SIDA, the birth control pill now became the central focus of the entire program, augmenting the use of the loop, if not replacing it outright. Moreover, the message was no longer entrusted to conventional forms of media—print, radio, and television—with an increasing emphasis placed on word of mouth. In other words, PPFK was now going to interact directly with the home, the apartment, and the village, sending its representatives to establish contact.

Mother's Clubs and New Approaches to Mass Media (1968–)

Mother's Clubs (ŏmoŏni hoe)

Although the FP program was generally regarded as a qualified success when the data began to accumulate in the mid- to late 1960s, many of the interested parties were concerned, especially with a significant turnover in loop acceptors by 1967. Even more troubling, while the vast majority of Koreans (88 percent) professed some knowledge of family planning, as measured in a 1966 KAP survey, fewer than one-third (27 percent) actually made the transition to putting the ideals of the program into practice.[93] In effect, many had learned of the program and approved of its basic principles, but they were unable or unwilling to adopt these practices in their daily lives. And, with respect to the loop, many women found the discomfort too much to endure, choosing to opt out, leaving the technology and the program behind after removal. If these women had figured primarily as "acceptors" in the first two to three years of the program (from 1964 to 1966), they now assumed an even more prominent role, the target of efforts designed to provide an alternative to the loop to retain a larger portion of the demographic.

In 1966, the possibility of including oral pills as an alternative to the loop first became a topic of discussion, although at this point it was not yet certain whether this meant a simple one-to-one substitution, with the pill now taking the place of prominence, or some other means of introducing the new item. In either case, the costs associated with making such a move were offset in part by a donation from SIDA, which had generously agreed to supply 1,300,000 oral pills to ensure a steady supply to the first 150,000 women anticipated for the project. As for their delivery, the decision in 1967 to proceed with the pill as a major component of FP meant that the program would have the opportunity of pursuing a different media strategy, one that would penetrate further than previous FP campaigns. Beginning in 1968, this measure took concrete form with the mobilization of a network of Mother's Clubs (*ŏmoŏni hoe*) designed to place representatives in direct contact with women, reaching even to remote areas.[94]

Like many practices borrowed by FP over the course of its program, the notion of mobilizing mothers as a specific group was not entirely new, and in fact similar groups conducted on an independent basis predated the 1968 start-up date.[95] The difference here lay in the comprehensive nature of the communication strategy, as well as the types of social science informing the campaign. FP had previously conducted its own door-to-door visits on a limited basis in selected areas, learning that follow-up visits and counseling tended to promote greater awareness and acceptance of new birth control technologies. The campaign was equally aware of the limited impact of radio and print advertisements in a country where the reach of media to rural areas was often ineffective, contingent on literacy and the ownership of appropriate technology (radio, TV) to receive updates. The Mother's Clubs combined the collective insights accumulated from several years of experience (from 1964 to 1968), placing a woman known to villagers in contact with those around her, effectively placing the campaign directly in the village in the form of a highly motivated individual.

The strategic use of existing social forms also promised to yield an effective campaign, as the Mother's Clubs would draw on the institution of a mutual exchange club, or *kye*, in which a group of Koreans formed a meeting group as a form of economic exchange. Each member contributed to a collective pool of funds, and then at regular intervals one or two members would be permitted to draw on the funds for their personal use, typically investment in a family business or some similar enterprise. This system of informal banking, regulated by the close-knit character of the community, translated well into other societies when Korean immigrants sought to establish their businesses abroad; here, too, the government could use the community to promote the birth control pill. Mother's Clubs would meet on a regular basis, organized around a prominent figure within the community, and while the gatherings were social in nature, birth control played a critical role in the setting.

The Mother's Clubs were an effective means of creating a far-reaching network, spanning the highest levels of the state to reach the most basic form of community, the village, and the ambitions driving the program required careful selection of members. The designated mothers typically required some basic level of education and literacy, having the skills necessary to maintain a reliable record of the distribution of birth control pills. The typical mother had already given birth to one or two children of her own, ranged in age from approximately her late twenties to early forties, and often had a husband who was himself an individual of some prominence in the village.[96] This is not to suggest that the clubs simply replicated the existing social hierarchy, but there certainly was some degree of overlap with existing social structures in assembling elements of the new program. After all, a similar idea had motivated informal birth control campaigns nearly a decade earlier, and now the idea was being put to use in a much more ambitious program.

The ambitions of the program were matched by participating international partners, who were eager to witness—and presumably to exploit to commercial advantage at a later date—the development of a growing base of pharmaceutical consumers in South Korea, focusing in particular on the birth control pill and related reproductive technologies.[97] As noted previously, Sweden provided a supply of pills during the initial stages through its developmental agency, SIDA, recognizing that the ROK lacked a reliable supply of the drug at this point.[98] This issue of supply proved critical, not just in terms of getting the distribution off the ground but also in terms of creating the appropriate perception of value for the pill. If the Mother's Clubs provided the means for channeling the pill to villages, it was not necessarily the case that the pill had to be supplied entirely free to "acceptors."[99]

In its literature, PPFK has characterized the distribution scheme as simply an attempt to create a "basic FP grass-roots channel" by mobilizing the "most active women" in villages to reach their immediate friends and neighbors.[100] These women distributed the birth control pills under their authority, while also housing a group forum for the discussion of issues and concerns relevant to this target demographic. In subsequent years, individual clubs undertook their own group projects, pooling their resources to promote community efforts of interest to members, even as FP remained the primary objective of the mobilization.[101] At the national level, the effort was coordinated by a smaller subset of "Pill Administrators and Community Organizers" (PACO), with one individual overseeing activity within a designated county, thereby adding an additional layer of oversight. From 1968 onward, as the emphasis shifted away from the loop (from 1964 to 1968) to promotion of the pill, IUD acceptance and retention would remain a vital secondary goal, as the extent of interaction with the population was now much closer.

Mass Communications and ROK Social Science

Although the 1966 KAP survey had captured a population with high exposure to the FP message, with a much lower yield in terms of the transition to practice, the reluctance to use the technologies became much more difficult after 1968. Information about the pill was now readily available from a local community member, a woman known to villagers, in keeping with emerging social science arguing that "acceptors" were much more likely to take seriously new information deriving from someone close to them. At the same time, media campaigns continued through print, radio, and television, targeted to reach large urban areas where new technologies made this style of promotion accessible. Also beginning in 1968, PPFK began to issue its own glossy publication aimed directly at women, *Happy Home* (*kajŏng ŭi pŏt*), a magazine designed specifically to promote the benefits of birth control and modern family living. Available to interested parties through the Mother's Clubs and placed strategically in FP clinics and doctor's offices, this publication took on the task of spreading the FP message. Moreover, the cover of each edition targeted specifically the *nongch'on* (rural residents) as a group, suggesting a regional and class element curiously absent from much of the scholarly literature.

If the primary aim of the clubs lay in the distribution of birth control, the actual means of delivery had to be more subtle, integrating the new technologies within the rhythms of daily life. The monthly meetings of an individual club, for example, might include a wide range of topics, including children's education, news and gossip from the community, and, by the early 1970s, the basic philosophy and motivations underlying the emerging New Village Movement.[102] In this kind of informal setting, women felt more comfortable discussing family planning; as club membership was strictly voluntary, there was no forced participation. With PPFK offering a small stipend—the equivalent of US$4.50—to underwrite the start-up and operating costs of the groups, Mother's Clubs soon began to expand the scope of their financial and collective activities, placing FP within a wider context of life improvement.

These group activities grew increasingly ambitious with time, building on the original conception of the *kye*, or mutual help association, to begin running the clubs on a limited self-sustaining financial basis. Within the village, a mother's club frequently conducted a rice-saving campaign or ran a village cooperative store, pooling its efforts to earn funds before ultimately returning the earnings to the community.[103] In agricultural areas, comprising much of rural South Korea, the clubs typically planted trees or leased their group labor out to local farmers, again using their earnings to improve the overall communal welfare. Some clubs even offered competition to local farmers through the purchase of a small lot of cattle or piglets, which were raised and sold by group members. The point is that FP had to fit within a larger scheme of village life if it was to be successful, and the Mother's Clubs, while officially overseen by the PPFK, encouraged a great deal of individual initiative and experimentation within the framework of these expectations.

Statistics, Scrutiny, and Social Science: Reconstructing the Rural

If the diversity of these activities stands beyond question, their impact on village women and their daily lives raises a comparable set of issues. Even as the Mother's Clubs offered an opportunity to gather together on a regular basis to discuss issues of concern to women, the clubs fell within the scope of state-sponsored activities. Furthermore, the second five-year plan, which ran from 1967–1971, brought in additional funds from USAID (U.S. Agency for International Development) and other international partners for social science research, meaning that the degree of scrutiny was increasing by the late 1960s and early 1970s.[104] In effect, the Mother's Clubs found themselves working within the intersection of powerful interests, with their agendas informed by state interests and their activities observed closely by a number of external actors, although to what effect remains an excellent question.

According to the many of the surveys conducted, Mother's Clubs were able to perform a wide range of functions, meaning that their actions were largely self-directed, even within the constraints imposed by the FP program.[105] To begin, the degree of scrutiny could never capture the geographical diversity and specificity of the individual groups distributed throughout the southern half of the peninsula, a point emphasized in a 1974 report published by Seoul National University. The data collection process was severely limited by access to many of these villages, still restricted to a single bus route by the turn of the decade. The chief function performed by the clubs, given this degree of autonomy, had to do with challenges to family dynamics and the act of decision making, with women coming to play an increasingly prominent role in running their own domestic affairs.

In particular, Korean women were no longer consulting their husbands, parents, or in-laws as frequently as in the past, according to many of the new surveys, choosing to act on their own.[106] More specifically, these broad trends, translated in terms of FP, meant that husbands and wives were talking far more frequently about family issues and making reproductive decisions as a couple, rather than as part of an extended family. This change, even if incremental, represented a dramatic reversal for rural areas in particular, generally more conservative in character and less likely to talk openly. From the perspective of participating international partners, the most important implication for these changing communication patterns had to do with gender, that is, the preference for sons both as the inheritor of the family line and as a means of support for the parents in old age.[107] The preference for sons had long been regarded as a major factor contributing to the popularity of spontaneous abortion and the phenomenon of multiple births, making it one of the major targets for FP in Asia.[108]

Along with the opening of communication lines, the process of opting to use reproductive technologies was eased by newer promotional materials accompanying their distribution, designed specifically for a population living and working with agriculture. The birth control pill, for example, was strategically associated with the rhythms of the day, and women were asked to take it according to a schedule set not by a clock (a specific hour) but by the movement of the sun (alternatively, sunrise or sunset).[109] The economic advantages accumulating from a smaller family size were translated into bags of rice or a highly valued commodity, rather than an abstract set of figures. If it is easy to read these materials a bit more critically in the present, it is useful to recall their aims, translating the goals and ambitions of family planning to meet the needs of rural communities, previously perceived to be largely outside the call of the state.

From a strictly managerial standpoint, the approach taken by PPFK materials at this time reflects the recognition that individual units of the clubs were effectively conducting their affairs independently, with oversight from the outside contingent on the initiative and good will of group leaders. Although officially the entire country was covered by Mother's Clubs from 1968 onward, this claim was likely more of a bureaucratic convention than a material reality: "There is no evidence that all of the number of the mother's clubs were organized in the year."[110] Likewise, although an external FP worker or PPFK representative might ideally attend a meeting during the early stages, this possibility, too, was increasingly unlikely with the rapid expansion of the system, which had to reach a target of 16,868 such groups.[111] Instead, the most frequent form of contact lay in monthly reports filed by group leaders, statistical portraits allowing national planners to capture a better picture of the realities of much of the country.

These reports formed a major part of the criteria by which individual groups were assessed, with "active" groups—as determined by the number of members, the frequency of their gatherings, and the visibility of group activities—being the goal. At the bureaucratic level, this type of connection between the state and the individual ensured a secondary level of record keeping, an additional measure of reliability. This might sound like redundancy, although we should recall that South Korea was, by the early 1970s, deeply committed to the Vietnam War, acutely concerned about its security after President Nixon's announcement of the "Guam Doctrine" in 1969, and soon to witness the suspension of its constitution (1972).[112] Along with the issue of scrutiny, these new measures were essential to a state apparatus still finding its way with rural residents, especially those outside the call of the state. Family planning remained the priority, but it also became an effective tool with which to evaluate the degree of responsiveness to related civic appeals.

In this bureaucratic use, the statistics gathered by the state became one of the primary means for reading the activities and character of the population. Organized as a scheme penetrating to the village level, family planning called for a mobilization at the province (*to*), county (*kun*), and town levels (*myŏn*), calling for close reporting at each of these levels and gradually building an infrastructure that could provide public health oversight to the entire country. When the Mother's Clubs offered a potentially liberating space, they also brought the state along with them by introducing it to many places where it had little access. We should not read the organizational scheme too skeptically but recognize its role in a South Korea with a heavily militarized culture.

Still, it is equally difficult to characterize family planning as entirely a top-down program dictated exclusively by state interests, as the participants would run the majority of the daily operations, especially the community activities. Within the villages, Mother's Clubs faced passive, and sometimes active, opposition, as men wondered what the women were doing in their monthly meetings.[113] Similarly, the commercial activities sponsored by Mother's Clubs offered a rare opportunity at empowerment, and the range of these activities expanded with the transition to a new decade.

The flexibility offered by the program ultimately has much to say about our primary concern here, the motivations explaining why South Korean women in particular, and men to a lesser extent, responded so enthusiastically to the state's call in the form of FP. The new types of bodily intervention, as uncomfortable as they might be, were perceived less as a form of interference than as a means of exerting control over one's life and family. The publicity campaigns and teaching strategies were careful to emphasize this point: FP was not a matter of a surgery, nor of the use of the loop, but of gaining a significant measure of personal autonomy. The transition from the extended family to the nuclear family proved appealing to a population who had experienced liberation (1945), division (from 1945 to 1948), and a civil war (from 1950 to 1953) within a span of less than a decade. In contrast to Taiwan, where the goal of retaking the mainland was tied to a perceived need for more children, South Korea never publicly linked its population aims to the elusive goal of unification with North Korea, selecting economic growth as its major priority instead.

A second major factor was the role of "normalization," the means by which the new interventions were carefully packaged and mobilized. As we have seen, the PPFK was highly conscious of its approach and began to use the Mother's Clubs (1968) only when a problem with the loop developed. Similarly, the turn from the late 1960s to the early 1970s witnessed the move toward a massive mobilization campaign known as the New Village Movement, an ambitious scheme aiming at nothing less than a complete overhaul of rural South Korea. For FP, this transition did not mean a loss of cultural power but rather a new placement as a campaign situated within a call for a broader set of transformations. To practice FP under these circumstances was not so much to be in compliance with the state as to take advantage of the opportunity to change one's life and immediate material surroundings.

With these positive, conjoined themes of self-concept and personal autonomy, it should not be surprising that the memory of FP in much of the historiography and in South Korean popular culture is not nearly as dark as one might expect. Andrei Lankov has a piece in his volume *The Dawn of Modern Korea* (2007) that touches briefly on some of the popular slogans associated with the FP movement; although he refers to the "then new and still much disputed policy," his effort captures just a momentary snapshot of the program. It is critical to recall that the numbers desired by the state continued to increase the pressure on target demographics even through the early 1980s, when South Korea was approaching a fertility rate below that of the replacement rate. To be more specific, the initial posters and commercials did not specify a number, whereas later campaigns called for three (3-3-35), then two, and eventually reached the conclusion that "even two is many," indicating a preference for a single child. Covering a period of nearly two decades (1964 through the early 1980s), even this brief summary should reinforce the rigidity and bureaucratic character associated with the FP scheme, even as it now appears almost comical.

Indeed, that is precisely how the makers of the film "*Chal sara pose!*" ("Let's Live Well!") (2006) chose to portray the period of the early 1970s, as a comic interlude prior to the arrival of the more familiar present. If the film distances itself from these events through a series of humorous vignettes, placing a female FP representative as the central figure, I want to suggest that it nevertheless captures much of the tension associated with its subject matter, as the legacy of FP still invites a good deal of controversy in South Korea today, and a great deal more needs to be said in terms of its effects as a regional and class-based intervention strategy, targeting rural populations. Recent efforts to interview FP workers and midwives represent only the beginning of this process, recognizing that the campaigns were far from neutral or natural and heavily interventionist in character, in this sense, placing them in a comparative developmental context, resembling the campaigns conducted in Indonesia and Singapore, not just those of neighbors Taiwan and Japan.

5 Taking Samples for the Nation: Historicizing the Biological Sample in the South Korean Antiparasite Campaigns, 1969–1995

Equating Rice with Life

In one of the most remarkable visual images created for the South Korean antiparasite campaigns (*kisaengch'ung pangmyŏl*) from 1969 to 1995 in the post–Korean War era, a young boy in a striped shirt fends off an oversized, menacing worm, nearly as large as as himself.[1] Holding a bowl of rice directly over his head, the boy desperately attempts to stave off his ravenous foe, which seeks to eat from the bowl, thereby depriving the young child of his daily allotment. The text placed below the image tells the viewer about a visceral connection between an individual's health and the need for constant vigilance in maintaining bodily integrity, invoking the claim, "My Health, My Responsibility."[2] Created at a time when South Korea remained extremely poor, less than two decades removed from the destructive experience of the Korean War, the poster serves as a palpable reminder of the poverty and associated social problems of the period, a time when reliable sources of housing remained scarce. Moreover, the image underscores what would become a central theme of the second decade of Park Chung Hee's rule (from 1969 through 1978), with the state sponsoring an extremely ambitious and aggressive series of public health initiatives designed to address the major sources of disease posing a threat to the nation.

Building Infrastructure through Previous Campaigns

The first two of these campaigns had an enormous impact in shaping the perceptions of South Koreans concerning their bodies and an appropriate role for the state in undertaking these new forms of public health intervention. Dating to the aftermath of the war, tuberculosis (*kyŏrhaek*) continued to represent a common health problem, so much so that one of the first postwar projects undertaken in the area adjacent to Severance Hospital—affiliated with Yonsei University since 1957—was a new hospital facility donated by the U.S. Eighth Army, devoted primarily to chest surgery.[3] As we saw in Chapter 3, this development held implications for the development of a program of surgical specialization at Seoul National University Hospital. Following this effort, family planning (FP) was adopted by the ROK state officially as of 1964, mobilizing an extremely aggressive set of interventions and accompanying reproductive technologies, including nationwide distribution of the Lippes loop (1964), the use of mobile transportation to reach rural areas (1966), and distribution of the birth control pill (1968), with this last method becoming the preferred choice by late in the decade.[4] In both cases, South Koreans encountered an extremely enthusiastic state apparatus, one eager to prove its effectiveness and organizational capacity in confronting existing health problems with a lengthy history.[5]

The third case, which had to wait until nearly the close of the decade to be addressed, concerned the uncomfortable presence of a wide range of parasites, a development often attributed to the frequent use of "night soil" as the primary source of fertilizer in an agricultural nation.[6] This pattern led to a cyclical scheme of infestation, with vegetables and other consumables serving to reintroduce the parasites into the bodies of South Koreans as a common feature of the diet. As the ROK government intensified its infrastructure efforts during the decade of the 1960s, including the construction of new sources of housing and refurbishment of the public water supply, it began to take a greater interest in tackling this problem, especially as infection rates were extremely high, with more than half of the population carrying some form of parasite—and frequently more than one, a phenomenon characterized as "polyparasitism"—according to the first national surveys conducted in the late 1960s.[7] Moreover, even as this issue was framed as a domestic concern, South Korea was engaged as a major actor in the Vietnam War from 1965 through 1973, with South Korean troops constituting a significant portion of the American "Many Flags" campaign, an effort to make conduct of the war appear more international in its scope.[8] Military medicine (*kunjin ŭihak*) and public health (*pogŏn*) thus began to intersect as areas of mutual interest when South Korean troops began to deploy to the Southeast Asian military theater as early as February 1965, with their health serving as a major source of concern.

Fortunately, the problem of creating a distribution network suited for public health needs was already underway with the FP campaigns, as the use of mobile transportation and local schools and clinics formed a critical part of the delivery system, a valuable move at a time when the majority of South Koreans continued to reside in villages.[9] Considerable effort had gone into the training of health care workers at the local level, with the FP campaigns requiring a large number of such professionals, here loosely defined, to insert the Lippes loop properly and to instruct both men and women concerning the basics of reproductive health.[10] Initially, the ROK lacked a sufficient number of doctors and nurses to meet its demand, with the majority of such professionals typically concentrated in its dense urban areas: Seoul, Taegu, and Pusan. For the FP campaigns, this problem led to a heavy reliance on the investment and the participation of concerned citizens as eager amateur participants, including the mobilization of Mother's Clubs beginning in 1968, enrolling women directly into the government effort. Although the antiparasite campaigns did not require nearly the same level of expertise in terms of providing health care at the local level, they did involve a similar type of appeal to the conscience of the nation, with individual participation mobilized as a deeply patriotic act of consent. In particular, the nation's schoolteachers became the central means through which the campaign conducted the majority of its collection activities, with success or failure determined by the criterion of high rates of sample collection.

The use of public schools in this fashion represented more than just a form of convenience, a means of access to large numbers of young children. South Korea's public schools, reopened in 1945 following the close of the war, were embraced enthusiastically as one of the few positive legacies dating to the American occupation of 1945 through 1948). Moreover, these institutions provided a crucible in which the ideals of citizens were formed; this factor, combined with a Confucian zeal for education, made the public schools central to the activity of rebuilding the nation. Placing the antiparasite campaigns here was motivated in part by ease of access, certainly, but the unusual encounter to come rapidly became a formative part of what it would mean to grow up as a young child in South Korea throughout much of this period.

The Persistence of the "Tropical"?

The continuities with existing health efforts proved lacking specifically in the area of the medical infrastructure necessary to execute the campaign, with

South Korea requiring the assistance of a subset of its international partners. Prominent among these were Japan, which, following the renewal of diplomatic relations in 1965, had begun to interact with the ROK at a number of different levels, investing anew in areas such as light industry. With respect to health care specifically, Japan had channeled much of its overseas development assistance (ODA) into its diplomatic community under the broad label of OTCA (Overseas Technical Cooperation Agency [Kaigai Gijutsu Kyōryoku Jigyōdan]), founded as of June 1962.[11] OTCA rapidly became the public face of a newer, emerging Japan within international circles, a decade removed from the experience of American occupation and, more important, signifying the good will of a nation becoming an economic powerhouse in the region. The organization thus provided a means to channel Japan's considerable technical and medical expertise to its neighboring countries, especially those still in the process of developing.

In the case of South Korea, the renewal of cooperation with Japan held ambivalent historical overtones, especially in the field of parasitology, where the Japanese had previously contributed a good deal through the academic program based at Keijo Imperial University.[12] Moreover, even with an intervening two decades, the field continued to represent a particular strength within Japan, a development that came as a surprise to many within OTCA. In a series of official reports published in the second half of the 1960s, OTCA even expressed surprise over the number of inquiries it was receiving for medical assistance, specifically with respect to the field of tropical medicine.[13] Japan simply did not regard itself as a "tropical" country, or so these reports would claim, leaving the question as to why other state actors might feel differently. In any case, Korea fell within a group of the top six recipients of Japanese medical and technical aid for this period, reinforcing the country's developmental status as the two nations restored their ties.

The group of nations falling within this cluster of Japanese aid recipients included a number of countries in Southeast Asia, a scenario that strengthens the perception of South Korea as continuing to hold the status of a developing nation. More specifically, the list encompasses Indonesia, Taiwan, India, the Philippines, and Thailand, with the ROK following closely at number six.[14] If the group members shared a pattern fairly typical for the period of 1966 through 1970 as one possessing mutual or overlapping "Free World" interests—with the possible exception of India, which was attempting to maintain a nonaligned position—it also hints at a colonial past scarcely two decades earlier, when Japan's empire had extended its reach. In other words, expertise in tropical medicine does not necessarily have to reflect a domestic concern; for Japan, such knowledge had likely derived from the management of its vast imperial enterprise, particularly those areas that it had colonized.

This chapter bases its set of questions on this earlier history, examining the legacy of tropical medicine and public health in South Korea as it was applied to two distinct, but nevertheless closely related, communities, the first including large segments of the domestic population (especially rural residents) and the second including younger male members of that same group as they traveled to work and fight in Vietnam. While the material aid received from Japan initially consisted of only a few items—a set of vehicles, analogous to those used in the FP campaigns for mobile transportation, along with some basic lab equipment, including microscopes—the ideas and practices borrowed ultimately played a much greater role in motivating the enthusiasm for taking biological samples in bulk, analyzing them, and ultimately reducing the rate of parasitic infection. In fighting the giant roundworm (*Ascaris lumbricoides*) in particular, KAPE (Korean Association for the Eradication of Pests), formed in 1964, channeled an older set of associations for campaigns directed against the presence of pests (rats, mice) within the surrounding area into a vigorous effort to cleanse the interior of the body, producing a set of healthy, disciplined young citizens and soldiers who could represent the nation proudly at home and abroad.

Transforming "Pests" into Parasites: Transforming the Object of Study (1959–1969)

With the public aware, and lines of communication undergoing strengthening during the FP campaigns, the government turned to the nation's public schools, using these facilities as its primary network through which to collect and examine stool samples on a mass scale for the presence of a wide range of parasites. The act of conveying a sample to school, typically wrapped in a piece of newspaper early in the campaign and later placed in an individual specimen bag provided for precisely this purpose, would become a familiar ritual to several generations of young South Koreans (from 1969 through 1988), with the contents to be deposited on the teacher's desk or in a large box located at the front of the classroom. We will return to the material implications of this practice in the following section, but for now a critical question remains: What does this activity have to do with the practice of medical work in South Korea?

If the provision of care through the FP efforts represented one of the first extensive interventions in reproductive health—bearing in mind previous efforts conducted during the Japanese colonial period—in South Korea, it is possible to suggest here that this activity, along with the antiparasite campaigns, played a significant role in the creation of a formative public health and biomedical network in South Korea over the long term.[15]

In using the term *biomedicine*, as distinguished from the more generic *medicine* or even *Western medicine*, my intent here is to call attention to the term's newly emerging range of associations, including both the material and the symbolic. Although the term was not yet in frequent usage in its Korean rendering—*saengmul ŭihak*, or literally, "biological medicine"—and would not be for some time (until at least the early 1980s), it is useful to introduce it here to emphasize the pace of rapid change taking place within the broader South Korean medical community.[16] Within the decade of 1961 through 1969, SNUH had adopted a new approach with respect to the bodies of its patients, taking far more samples and performing many more autopsies, indicating some (if limited) use of the human body as an object of research. Similarly, the FP campaigns, while concerned primarily with reproductive health and the demographics of population, had offered another opportunity to engage in work where health policy and the life sciences would intersect.

Saengmul ŭihak, or the "medicine of living things," connotes at least three clusters of associations, the first being the intersection of the life sciences (*saengmulhak*/biology) with some notion of the broader practice of medicine. In its Korean usage, moreover, the term further reflects a Japanese understanding of the Western form of biomedical practice, with the etymology indicating the likely pattern of the movement of knowledge. In addition, the term implies a systemic or ecological approach, that is, the placement of the human within a larger community of living organisms and the corresponding attempt to research and understand the body at a higher level. In contrast to physiology (*saengnihak*), which has a similar derivation, the term suggests the interaction of humans and other creatures and, more important, an attempt to understand these relationships. In this respect, it is not unreasonable to treat these early efforts as a very early stage for subsequent bioscience work, even if oriented very differently from a strictly scientific point of view.

This last point has to remain speculative, of course, as the much publicized biotech effort taking place in South Korea since 1997 clearly reflects a very different set of priorities.[17] More important to the present discussion is retaining the broad notion of a systemic understanding during the campaigns, the attempt to place the human within the context of the surrounding environment, with that setting including the presence of other creatures. This idea fits well with the mobilization of parasitology that soon took place, as the field involves understanding any number of microorganisms and their placement within a larger ecosystem. Parasitology, in other words, involves more than the mere elimination of such creatures for the sake of human convenience and aims that the parasitic organisms be understood in relation to their host organism. If this language appears new for South Korea at this time, in fact it was not, as an earlier generation of Japanese scholars had frequently made similar observations about the peninsula dating to the late 1920s and early 1930s as part of the mobilization for war.[18]

Strictly speaking, South Korea and the Korean peninsula lie well outside the zone described by the two tropics—the Tropic of Cancer and the Tropic of Capricorn—meaning that tropical medicine does not necessarily represent a natural fit as an applied field of study. However, the category of the tropical being applied to the region begins to make sense when we consider the ambitions of the Japanese empire spanning the late nineteenth through the mid-twentieth centuries. Taiwan, in particular, was on the receiving end of a great deal of attention devoted to this kind of study, and Japan expanded to encompass large parts of southeast Asia during the later war years, from 1942 through 1945, even as this imperial vision would ultimately prove untenable. The appeal to OTCA, which Japan professed not to understand, arguably reflects this earlier history, with newer forms of developmental assistance representing a subsequent iteration of an earlier form of colonial medicine.

Just because the Japanese held a set of beliefs about the Korean peninsula as part of its empire does not necessarily mean that South Korean actors thought and experienced the same thing several decades later, of course. However, that the "tropical" might present an ongoing problematic does make sense in light of the (limited) number of elite Koreans who had trained under the imperial system of medical education. By the time of the early to mid-1960s, moreover, the issue was on their minds, especially as a convenient index of comparative development, a point of contrast serving to distinguish the developing nation from its surrounding neighbors. Prior to traveling to Vietnam, the prevailing assumption was that South Korean forces would be at risk from disease and parasitic infection in Southeast Asia, requiring that a baseline survey be taken prior to departure. Similarly, the separation between the urban and the rural within the nation itself suggested very different developmental trajectories, invoking the need for some type of survey conducted on a large scale.

The language with which this perceived line of difference was formulated may not have been codified according to the academic tradition of tropical medicine (*yŏltae ŭihak*), but it did connote a much longer range of associations with the handling of pests. In an agricultural nation, Koreans were familiar with the problem of bringing in the harvest and storing it safely by stowing it under carefully controlled conditions. Similarly, Koreans were no doubt familiar with living with farm animals, especially bovine creatures, and knew many of the diseases common to these creatures.[19] In fact, the veterinary program at Seoul National University had provided training to several Korean experts during the Minnesota Project, and we will return to this point shortly. For now, the key is recognizing that the antiparasite campaigns, for all of their systemic fervor, were not so much "new" as a reformulation of prior practices, an update to more traditional campaigns designed to eliminate pests, especially mice and rats, creatures eager to feed on quantities of stored grains, from human surroundings.

Rats, Worms, and History: Mobilization Prior to the Antiparasite Campaigns (1954–1969)

Campaigns against such creatures have a lengthy history within the broader East Asian context, and certainly Mao's China remains famously linked to its fervent desire to limit the impact of pests (rats, flies, mosquitoes, and sparrows) post-1949.[20] For South Korea specifically, the need to historicize this type of activity has less to do with determining a single point of origin and more with establishing a strong contrast between the antipest campaigns and the subsequent, more biomedical, activity directed against parasites. Rats, in particular, would receive a great deal of attention from the start of the Park Chung Hee period (from 1961 to 1979), with specific days devoted to catching and eliminating their presence. As evidence of a successful catch, schoolchildren would sometimes be asked to provide a certain number of the animal's tails, which would attest to their faithful participation. As with the anxiety associated with sampling, some schoolchildren proved unsuccessful at this, necessitating that some other form of evidence be brought to school.

The initial burst of enthusiasm associated with these campaigns would date to the first few weeks following the seizure of power after the May 16, 1961, coup, covering a month-long interval from May 25, 1961, to June 25.[21]

The proximity of this particular campaign to the inception of a new government almost certainly reinforces the idea of a mobilization undertaken specifically for ideological purposes conjoined with nation-building instincts, demonstrating the effectiveness of a new style of leadership, "cleaning house" both materially and symbolically. In this and subsequent Park-era campaigns, the activity would generally be authorized under the sponsorship of one of the ministries responsible for agriculture, most frequently the Agriculture and Fisheries Department (*Nongsusanbu*). The point here is less one of ascertaining a specific source for this activity, an effort to define the activity of rat catching via periodization, and, instead, recognizing that it was used at critical moments to channel and redirect popular forms of enthusiasm.

For precisely this reason, there remain many wonderful, apocryphal stories from the period of young students crafting a set of tails out of some similar, stringy material, with the offering to be handed in at school. The composition in this case might include fragments of a piece of leather, or anything similar that might be crafted to approximate the shape of a rat tail. And if a majority of these stories date to the early Park period, there is little doubt that antipest activity may be traced backward, covering the tenure of Syngman Rhee and perhaps even earlier. Rather than a firm date, this activity suggests a much longer cluster of associations, capturing the deeply rooted anxiety directed at natural phenomena that exceed human control, bringing trouble to an agricultural community. And if rats would receive a great deal of attention, the activities designed to speed their demise appear less systemic, aiming simply at killing them.

To expand on this last point, it is not difficult to locate public displays from this period, with a significant part of the pedagogical intent involving public education and awareness, recognizing the danger posed by rats to the food and grain supply.[22] Along with this, area residents would be asked to put out rat poison at regular intervals, with specific days named as designated points, further reinforcing a desired change to public behavior. As thorough as these campaigns often were, though, they did not involve any form of intervention to the human body, nor were they systemic in the sense of the creation of a new infrastructure. I want to suggest that while the antiparasite campaigns represent continuity with this earlier enthusiasm, they were distinct at the same time, requiring the construction of a new research community in parallel with the campaigns.

Defining a Professional Community

Falling roughly at the midpoint of the period comprising the 1961 campaign directed against rats and the 1969 start of the national antiparasite effort would be the formation of a society devoted to addressing the problem, with KAPE organized as a formal body in 1964. Although KAPE hoped to include public outreach as part of it original mission, its composition reflected a much more elite, limited membership at the outset, including among its members the select few who had studied academic parasitology either in South Korea or, ideally, at a university abroad. Rather than making a discontinuity argument here, I include KAPE as part of a series of incremental changes, one reflecting the earlier enthusiasm for handling pests, even while channelling this energy in the direction of a more professional, scientific set of founding principles. That is, KAPE aimed for an even more ambitious set of strategies in attacking its designated targets, naming a collective category of parasites as its target and seeking their control and elimination on biological grounds.

In linking together these distinct moments—1961, 1964, and 1969—it should be clear that the amount of activity devoted to pests and parasites was intensifying even before South Korea became involved in the Southeast Asian conflict (1965), suggesting that the motives informing the actors were likely diverse in character. In the earliest of these campaigns (1961), along with a nation-building impulse, Park and his followers determined that simply appealing to South Korean society was a good idea, regardless of the object. The formation of KAPE, taking place a few years later in 1964, witnessed the convergence of a set of state interests with the corresponding drive for professionalization among a select group of academics and policymakers. The two sets of actors found that they could further their mutual ambitions by working together. Moreover, this joint activity could be directed at improving the position of South Korea with respect to its neighbors, as the nation was becoming increasingly visible.

The actors directing the campaigns within the field of parasitology saw their career opportunities enhanced, given the opportunity to take their work from the classroom to the field, with the domestic context representing the first site from 1964 through 1969. At least officially, academic parasitology in South Korea dates to the post–Korean War period, constituting an explicit denial of any connection or lingering influence deriving from the period of Japanese colonial rule. At Seoul National University, for example, the Department of Parasitology and Tropical Medicine locates its formation to 1954, with

Dr. Byung Seol Seo, soon a contributing figure both at KAPE and in the studies of ROK soldiers based in Vietnam, playing the role of the central actor. Dr. Seo, along with several of his younger Korean colleagues, had the opportunity to study abroad, in his case as a participant in the Minnesota Project (1955), thereby exposing him to American models of parasitology along with his previous training.

With his period of study abroad in Minneapolis, Dr. Seo also holds great interest because of his formative role within South Korean parasitological circles, and he was present at the formation of the Korean Society of Parasitology (1959), along with a number of other figures who have appeared in these chapters. For example, both Dr. Kwon E. Hyock and Dr. Yang Jae-Mo, though better known for their prominent roles in South Korean public health and family planning, also attended the January 1959 meeting at which Dr. Seo and his colleagues assembled their new fraternity. According to one historical account, this intersection should not be surprising, as Korean academia was extremely small at this time, frequently bringing together actors across a range of fields.[23] In fact, only a quarter of those attending had formal training in parasitology, with five individuals specializing in medical parasitology and two others having a specialty in veterinary parasitology.

Rather than separate themselves into their distinct subfields, the relatively small numbers of medically trained elites in South Korea tended to share their activities as a collective, motivated by a sense of collegiality and in many cases, out of basic necessity, sharing a limited pool of resources. The seven parasitologists present at the first meeting therefore found themselves complemented by a diverse group of twenty-one additional actors. These individuals had training in a cluster of related fields, including the clinical sciences, preventive medicine, medical bacteriology and biology.[24] Along with the formative program at Seoul National University, there was a comparable program in parasitology taking shape at Yonsei University (1958), headed by Dr. Chin-Thack Soh.[25] Dr. Soh, like his colleagues from Seoul National, was fortunate to have had the opportunity to spend time abroad in the United States, in his case completing a tour of study at Tulane University.

Along with the new motivation supplied by study abroad, the Korean War served as a major source of innovation and change in parasitology, bringing both professionals and ordinary Koreans into regular contact and unwanted familiarity with parasites. As during the occupation, U.S. forces would rely heavily on DDT as a stopgap remedy, dusting large numbers of Korean villagers and their children in the hopes of limiting the spread of typhus. During this time, parasitology and public health were closely tied to military medicine, not surprisingly, and this relationship would translate well in the Korean context, applying public health and medicine in a crisis situation. In the postwar period (from 1954 to 1961), we must therefore recognize ROK military medicine as one of the critical patrons driving growth in the field, along with its more exclusive academic counterpart.

Together, the academy and military medicine would help to transform South Korea domestically and regionally, targeting a select group of parasites for further study, developing a deeper understanding in the process of strategizing and recommending methods of control. Of these new objects, we will focus the discussion here on the giant roundworm, or *Ascaris*, as this target would receive the majority of attention in the campaigns. And if there were no direct, material links between contact with OTCA and earlier models of Japanese pedagogy dating to the colonial era, it is nonetheless fair to consider this period as one of reintegrating the Korean academy into first the regional and next into the world academic communities, selecting from an eclectic range of models in developing its own knowledge style and forms of practice.

In reaching out to a domestic constituency first and later its close regional partners, South Korea was acutely aware of the significance of perception, using the antiparasite campaigns as a means to compare itself to others. In this respect, the second of these two audiences, especially with the growing importance of Southeast Asia by 1965, presented a practical problem requiring the judicious use of these new forms of expertise. Thailand had been a close partner since its intervention in the Korean War, and soon (in December 1965) Hyundai Construction would send its engineers and planners to begin work on the Pattani–Naratiwat highway (from 1965 to 1968), a construction effort financed by the World Bank. In the Vietnam context, similarly, it was not just South Korean troops, but also large numbers of support personnel, who would travel to the region and provide infrastructural support to back the American war effort with the construction of airstrips, highways, and dredging. Hyundai Construction would become one of the largest contractors working for the Americans in the field, learning how to secure bids and carry out large construction projects under difficult conditions.

The conjoined potential of revenue and learning opportunities for Hyundai was only one of the new possibilities made available in this context and, for the parasitologists like Dr. Seo, the chance to develop their regional and international partnerships was even more valuable. The Korean War had brought South Korea attention as a partner and a postwar aid recipient, transforming what had been a site previously defined by its Japanese contacts into a much more diverse place. Even as American actors would now play a prominent role, they represented only one subset of the partners wanting to exchange ideas and practices. Dr. Seo, for example, would soon become involved in WHO (the World Health Organization), with the postwar growth of international health providing numerous opportunities to develop new transnational relationships. For South Korea, this meant not only Northeast Asia but now increasingly the southeast, including Thailand and the Philippines.

As an index of comparative development, parasitology thus held the potential to reach out to the smallest village in a rural area as well as to other nations, especially those where large numbers of South Koreans might be traveling. The language with which these results would be framed needed to be careful, of course, so as not to arouse regional sensibilities, with this observation perhaps even more relevant than in the domestic context. And if the ambitions of a small group of trained professionals led the campaigns, a much larger set of hands would be needed as a complement, individuals to process and analyze the samples to be collected on site at the nation's public schools. Here OTCA helped with the setup of infrastructure, and South Korea needed to make changes to its own pedagogy to create a new category of workers.

Sample Collection and Analysis: Sampling Becomes "Normal" (1969–)

Herein lies the strength of the organizational scheme on which the campaigns depended, the decision to reach out through the public schools, relying on primary, middle, and high school teachers to stand in as agents of the state during the process of collection. The approach required twice yearly collection and inspection of samples for nearly two decades (from 1969 to 1988) at six-month intervals, with virtually the entire population under the age of eighteen receiving attention. As attendance at public schools was mandatory and enforced by law, the system possessed an effective means to deal with its target demographic, those who might otherwise miss out on the reach of public health. In addition, there were related campaigns focusing on select populations (for example, military) distinct from the school campaigns. In brief, attending school throughout this period meant that the donation of one's stool sample would become a familiar, if not necessarily comfortable, biannual ritual.

While remaining cautious about making culture-specific generalizations, it is worth pausing here for a moment to revisit the issue of the sampling process itself, which in fact required a great deal of public outreach, as did the entire program, especially in terms of eliciting participation. In a study conducted late in the second half of the 1950s, Dr. Jae-Mo Yang, then affiliated with Severance Hospital, had compared the preferences of his Korean patients to "shoppers," that is, private individuals holding no special "brand allegiance" to either Western medicine or traditional practice and instead choosing an appropriate form of treatment as circumstances best suited them. This remark should serve as a palpable reminder that Korean practitioners (TKM) continued to outnumber their Western-trained counterparts in the aftermath of World War II and played a critical role in maintaining subsistence health care, encouraging a particular set of attitudes toward the body and diet.

The Body and Biomedicine

At around the same time, American doctors serving in Seoul as part of the Minnesota Project (from 1954 to 1962) noted that the Seoul National University hospital seldom took tissue samples or specimens in the course of conducting its routine business.[26] In the context of the time, this trend—assuming the observation is an accurate one—likely had a great deal to do with the economics of the situation, specifically the lack of refrigeration and laboratory facilities for analysis at the hospital, especially in the aftermath of the Korean War. Regardless, the American team made this point one of their quantitative goals for the reform of clinical medicine, actively encouraging and tracking the number of samples taken. The drive then went on to mobilize the autopsy as a related tool for encouraging further analysis, with Korean interns and physicians receiving a small cash payment in the event of persuading a family to permit an autopsy on the body of a loved one. Again, while remaining cautious about drawing any conclusions here, it is safe to say that the clinical culture of South Korean medicine at this time included less frequent contact with the physical body than did its counterparts in other national settings, as this theme emerges repeatedly in reports issued in conjunction with the project.

For the autopsy specifically, respect for the integrity of the body often stemmed from religious views, with cremation reserved for certain cases, generally suicides or those without a family. The introduction of cremation as an efficient, modern form of burial and disposal therefore met with considerable resistance when it first appeared during the colonial period. In retrospect, these concerns seem quite minor, as more than half of South Koreans now undergo cremation, given the lack of available land and related environmental concerns. At the same time, we need to recognize that the transition point for this activity dates to precisely the period under discussion here (from 1953 through the present), with urbanization and the move to apartments creating radical changes in South Korean living habits. This type of change deserves mention here as it reinforces the notion that medical intervention in the body, whether in life or death, represents a relatively recent phenomenon in South Korea, and one that would typically be accompanied with discomfort.

For many South Koreans, the encounter with the state in the form of these campaigns constituted one of the first experiences of biomedicine, along with related health campaigns dating to this period. For its part, the state also needed to prepare a means of gathering and analyzing the samples, identifying the positive cases in an efficient and timely matter. This was no small matter in a country with a very limited scientific community and with a medical community based largely in a few urban areas. The government had to create a new category of employment to meet the need, medical technicians who would require specialized education to the *chŏnmun hakkyo* level (two years of training following graduation from high school), before applying for a license. As a group, these individuals constituted the core of the sampling system, examining thousands of samples nationwide, representing the baseline criteria to determine the presence or absence of parasites.

The creation of this new category of expertise raises the accompanying question of the handling procedures by which the samples were analyzed. Here, assistance from OTCA again proved invaluable, as South Korea was simply not equipped to perform even this basic level of lab work with its current facilities. First, and most important, the Koreans followed the model of the Kato "thick smear" technique, whereby a piece of cellophane tape was applied to each sample, with the resulting adhesion of stool material applied to a glass slide.[27] The placement of a cover slip for microscopic analysis completed the process, with the cover slip held in place by the intervening layers of sample material, as well as through the application of light pressure supplied with a handheld stamp.[28] Although this procedure sounds more than a bit improvised and even a bit crude, it was designed specifically for the field conditions of rural South Korea and similar types of outdoor locations (Southeast Asia), and it hardly constituted a delicate set of handling rules for samples such as one might expect of controlled laboratory conditions. Rather, this approach was designed for processing of samples in bulk, with the motivation of getting either a positive or negative reading, rather than aiming at a precise count of the number and variety of parasites.

Much of the hardware for the project derived from a Japanese source, Elmo, Ltd., a Nagoya-based optics firm, with the company furnishing a range of instruments for analysis and lab work, as well as for pedagogy. For the former, microscopes of varying power gave the Koreans a reliable set of tools with which to examine samples on a large scale, making a relatively quick and easy determination regarding the presence of parasite eggs. Elmo also provided centrifuges and related types of equipment to enable their South Korean colleagues to establish the required conditions for a central set of readymade labs as the samples were gathered and pooled for analysis. Equally important, the South Korean government emphasized public outreach as a major component of its campaign, supplying lessons to the public in soliciting their cooperation. Much of this equipment, too—ranging from educational filmstrips and projectors to tape recorders—came from Elmo, although it is not clear whether the firm supplied only the hardware or whether it assisted with the audio and video content as well.

This last point should not be taken as a mere reminder of the Japanese presence but, rather, as an effort to emphasize the resurgence of the role played by Japanese technology, equipment, and models of practice in shaping regional practice following the restoration of diplomatic relations in 1965. Moreover, highlighting this point is useful because I want to touch on the proximity—both materially and temporally—between South Korean public health campaigns and the development of subsequent medical practice. That is, conditions in a developmental state were such that this type of large-scale field effort represents, at least in part, the origins of a domestic tradition of health and medical research, along with the Minnesota Project. Most Koreans did not become familiar with the process of allowing their bodies to be examined regularly and permitting the taking of samples until the promotion of these national efforts beginning in the late 1960s. In material terms, this work could be accomplished only by importing the majority of the equipment, and a new category of technician had to be created to accommodate the need for trained eyes to examine specimens in bulk.

The return portion of the cycle also leaned heavily on international partners, as mentioned earlier, with the medicine to be dispensed coming from a range of sources. Two issues here deserve special mention: the problem of intellectual property and the types of social distinction to be created through the treatments provided, whether coincidental or not. South Korea had no research tradition sufficient to meet all of its own chemical needs and to distribute them through a domestic pharmaceutical industry. It did, however, have a chemical community sufficiently skilled at taking and analyzing samples of imported pharmaceuticals before rendering comparable versions of these to be synthesized locally and distributed on a mass scale. In some cases, the South Korean government was able to persuade its partners either to donate the drugs outright or to provide a substantial discount on the rights, thereby providing the remedy to residents at low cost. In others, however, the Korean Association for Health Promotion acknowledges that legal protections were ignored in the drive to provide appropriate medications to South Korean residents, adopting an attitude that the act of copying a compound was justified in the national interest.

If the act of taking samples was unfamiliar, the response to the distribution of medicine met with a range of responses. For one, the compounds available at the initial stages were not always effective, and there remain numerous apocryphal accounts of those who had ingested a compound in the belief that it would kill pests, only to expel live parasites from the gastrointestinal tract. KAPE also reports that some resisted passively, accepting the medication offered but later disposing of it, only pretending to swallow. These types of behaviors are familiar in any large public health campaign and so could be dealt with in turn, but what was more problematic was the type of implicit social and class categories being created as an indirect consequence of the campaigns. At first, the chemotherapy was performed on a mass scale—labelled a "mass control" program—with all students receiving the drugs, operating on the assumption that safety and prevention were the major concern. As the numbers began to dwindle after more than a decade of attention, however, the project shifted in emphasis, dispensing only to those who had tested positive.

Although the logic behind this change in approach is justifiable in terms of economy and efficiency, the effects on those individuals receiving a positive diagnosis remain one of the more uncomfortable legacies of the program. As the numbers decreased rapidly by the early to mid-1980s, and especially as the twice-yearly ritual of submitting a sample began to disappear late in that same decade (by 1988), the stigma associated with a positive diagnosis would become more visible. Children knew that when a few classmates were called aside by the teacher that these individuals likely had a problem with parasites; in a very real sense the antiparasite campaigns redefined what it meant to grow up "rural" in South Korea as determined by a specific set of health criteria. Whereas once this definition could be regarded as simply a geographical designation, one reinforced through the lens of Japanese colonialism, it now became a label assigned by an individual's own government and, more specifically, his or her own school, based on the intersection of highly specific economic and health indicators. Although the "Miracle of the Han," the mythic rise of the South Korean economy beginning in the mid-1960s, remains a powerful story endorsed by the ROK state, the reality is that much of this growth was confined to a narrow corridor running from the urban northwest (Seoul) to the southeast (Pusan), encompassing the major cities while bypassing adjacent areas.

As a form of public health, the antiparasite campaigns formed a major part of this success narrative; in fact, this is the way that many of the participants have chosen to remember their roles. However, the campaigns also played a critical part in dramatically reshaping attitudes and material practices surrounding the body, especially in terms of the growing acceptability of intervention by a health professional, even in the apparently minor task of taking and analyzing a stool sample. Again, we need to recall that South Korea was a thoroughly militarized state for much of this time, with compulsory military service for males, an active role in the conduct of the Vietnam War, and the suspension of its constitution in late 1972, the period of Yushin rule (*yusin sidae*). Along with the antiparasite campaigns, the national family planning effort (from 1964 through the early 1980s) left few homes untouched, with a series of birth control technologies distributed to women and men encouraged to seriously consider the possibility of voluntary sterilization, with material incentives (better access to new apartments) for those consenting to the surgery.[29]

Following on this, ROK military culture has become a subject of interest in recent years, especially through the work of Vassar sociologist Seungsook Moon and her notion of "militarized modernity"—with this term connoting the close relationship between the style of construction and engineering learned in the ROK military and its implications for civilian life, along with the close personal relationships formed during service leading to long-term gendered ties in the corporate sector—and it is only appropriate that the military would serve as a vehicle for the distribution of a particular style of medicine.[30] Although both Moon and diplomatic historian Gregg Brazinsky have emphasized the ROK military as a civil institution for the building of the state apparatus, to date scholars have not looked at military medicine (*kunjin ŭihak*) as a related component of this "civilizing" process on behalf of the state.[31] With mandatory conscription, and with military public health arguably beginning as early as 1946, even prior to the formation of a state per se, military service played a hugely influential role in exposing South Korean males to the expectations and norms of a common culture of modern medicine, defining a "healthy" soldier in terms of specific criteria, thereby promoting the ideals identified with the new nation.

Moreover, the possibility of employing medicine in this fashion was not entirely a new idea, as the intense encounter with American military medicine had produced a rapid series of transformations within South Korean medicine during the Korean War, later to be accompanied by the work of the Minnesota Project. Working side-by-side with American colleagues in the challenging conditions of field hospitals, not to mention the better-equipped facilities situated in the rear areas, safely away from combat, South Korean doctors and nurses had received the equivalent of a postgraduate course in American military medicine. As we saw in Chapter 3, this accelerated learning curve contributed to the ambitious scale of the postwar rehabilitation efforts, but for now the point is that ROK military medicine became a means of establishing a style of uniformity, processing Korean males of all types at the intake point, with the explicit goal of producing a particular type of soldier on the other end.

Parasites and Vietnam: *Kunjin ŭihak* ("Military Medicine"), 1965–1973

Within the history of medicine, there is a lengthy tradition of utilizing "captive" populations—referring here to prisoners, colonial subjects, and military conscripts—as part of the process of testing and perfecting new remedies and pharmaceuticals through clinical trials. South Korean soldiers would prove no exception to this trend, appearing in the *Korean Journal of Parasitology* as early as 1963, in this case in conjunction with a baseline study of the distribution of parasites among their members.[32] With mobilization for the Vietnam conflict beginning early in 1965, even prior to America's formal commitment to the war, South Korean forces were exposed to a wide variety of environmental conditions, placing their health and well-being at risk.[33] The climate, humidity, and physical topography of Vietnam exposed these soldiers to a wide range of disease conditions, including not only parasites but also the prospect of tropical disease, with malaria representing a potent threat.[34] Moreover, their diet needed to change substantially, as many of these soldiers, subsisting previously on a diet based heavily on rice, were now asked to eat processed foods for at least part of the time, including whatever canned or packaged meals might be available in the improvised conditions of the field.

In their previous encounters with the American military, South Koreans had discovered with surprise that their own country looked different when seen through foreign eyes. A fascinating side story to the Korean conflict involves the impact of disease factors, and the accompanying perception that the Korean peninsula was a site rich with the prospect of illness. In addition to the problems detailed in Chapter 3, the American military would become deeply concerned with hemorrhagic fever (hanta virus) and malaria, with the former leading to any number of problems for the kidneys. While never labelling South Korea as "tropical," Americans certainly regarded conditions on the peninsula as perilous, and they developed a fresh sense of the acute need for maintaining hygiene. To return to Vietnam, it is difficult to know how much of this discourse would have filtered back to the South Koreans, but it is fair to speculate that similar sets of disease concerns would be mapped reciprocally onto the Vietnamese population.

Within South Korea, the image of the war as one based on anticommunist activity made for a popular mobilization, and a number of historians have pointed out the ways this venture would serve to modernize the ROK military through exposure to new combat conditions and through a dramatic overhaul of their equipment and training via the terms of MAP (Military Assistance Program), overseen by the United States.[35] This was a war of medical modernization as well, even more so than the Korean War, with college students participating in domestic blood drives to provide a sufficient supply for the front.[36] As the war dragged on, the return of the deceased, those killed in action, also brought home the tangible realities of death, as respects had to be paid and loved ones buried. Again, these activities were not new per se, but the Vietnam War provided the first such collective mobilization for South Korea as a nation since the divisive Korean War a decade earlier and, in this respect, offered an opportunity for redemption through collective action. This was a chance to mold new soldiers on behalf of the nation, and, in the course of their training, their bodies and health would be very much at issue.

Tropical Medicine in the Korean Context: Identifying Populations

Tropical medicine has an unusual background in South Korea's medical historiography in that it did not originate with a colonial venture undertaken on behalf of the nation. In part, it represented a continuation of the Japanese presence, especially centered on the work of controversial figure Dr. Harujiro Kobayashi, dating to the imperial university period, even as a good deal of the local historiography has aimed at reducing his presence as a contributing factor. In the decade prior to involvement in Vietnam, at least three professors from Seoul National University, among them Dr. Byung Seo Seol (1955) and Dr. Rim Han Jong (1959), had spent periods of study at the University of Minnesota, familiarizing themselves with more recent and emerging American models of practice. By the early 1960s, parasitology and tropical medicine had assumed the form of a growing practice, with the primary aim of studying and treating disease vectors specific to the Korean peninsula. It was Dr. Rim specifically who had published on the issue of parasites within the South Korean military, underscoring a growing interest at establishing a broad portrait of the problem prior to a consideration of possible remedies.

As the nation prepared for the Vietnam venture, the infrastructure required to support such an ambitious project effectively brought medicine along with it, as South Korean doctors saw a opportunity to undertake research in the field. Of great interest was the possibility of conducting comparative work, even as the sets of motivations informing this impulse remained somewhat murky. At least implicitly, and sometimes quite openly, South Korean researchers sought to establish a pattern of differences between their own troops and the habits and lifestyle of the Vietnamese population. J. K. Kim, for example, would report on the dwellings of Vietnamese villagers, noting the composition of such structures and, more specifically, closely observing the lack of a separate latrine or kitchen in the home, an obvious point of concern from a public health standpoint.[37] Subsequent studies commented extensively on the toilet habits of Vietnamese—"people defecate around household, door yard, road side, or in the fields"—and on the length of their fingernails, with these minute differences accumulating to form a portrait of perceived ethnic and cultural difference.[38]

These images of difference, whether real or constructed, should not minimize the very genuine prospect of confronting the problem of disease in the field. The majority of South Korean troops could expect to spend at least a year in Vietnam during their rotation in country, throughout which they would be exposed to a number of new and unfamiliar disease vectors. If the presence of parasites offered one point of comparison, a subject to which we shall return, a second and equally critical issue centered on addressing the possible spread of malaria, something with which Koreans were already familiar. At the time, malaria continued to represent a minor but irritating problem in South Korea; more specifically, this claim refers to the tertian form of malaria. The quartan and tropical forms of malaria, on the other hand, were considered to be problems tied to a highly specific population, narcotics addicts, because of their frequent use of needles in unsafe and unhygienic conditions. These temporal labels refer to the periodicity of the fever cycle, meaning a recurrence of approximately every three (tertian) to four days (quartan), suggesting that only the less severe forms were linked directly to South Korea. Again, we can see here the basis for a comparison—contrasting an endemic condition with an infection deemed to derive from the use of illegal narcotics—even as the primary focus rested on the issue of how to handle malaria under battlefield conditions.

Even as tropical malaria was still considered an "exotic" disease—one not frequently seen on the Korean peninsula—by South Korean specialists, they had to begin addressing it as a regular feature of life in Vietnam, especially as it had an impact on a large number of their troops. Previous work in the area, including publications by Byung Seol Seo nearly a decade earlier (1959), had acknowledged the existence of a limited number of cases in the ROK, with an association made between the condition and the improper use of hypodermics.[39] In Vietnam, on the other hand, the number of cases that affected ROK forces appeared almost simultaneously with the arrival of large numbers of troops, with the greatest concentration of studies published in the first two years of the South Korean military presence (between 1965 and 1967).[40] The majority of these publications were advisory in scope, treating the problem primarily as one of vector control, seeking to limit exposure and to eradicate mosquito populations whenever possible. At the same time, the problem allowed for the opportunity to begin comparative work and, more important, to perfect techniques necessary to perform sample analysis and collection, in this case looking specifically at the plasmodium vivax (less severe) and plasmodium farciparum (more severe).

Dr. Seo's study of malaria patients among ROK troops, published in 1970, touches on this last point without necessarily making explicit the critical importance of the ability to perform this kind of delicate biological work.[41] That is, we have previously seen the relatively crude forms of equipment and training available for analysis at the beginning of the antiparasite campaigns, with numerous partners, Japan in particular, helping to bring South Korea up to speed. In the case of malaria, Dr. Seo and his collaborators report that they performed the work of analysis on their own, although details are not provided concerning the material conditions under which this was accomplished. What we do learn is that "thick slides" were used to establish the presence and density of the various forms of the plasmodium, with "thin slides" later used for a closer look at the morphology and size of the different types of bacteria. The samples were taken from ROK troops infected with malaria, those who had been evacuated from the battlefield due to the severity of their condition.

At least indirectly, Seo's article suggests an ability to handle the samples and analysis on an independent basis, although it is fair to speculate whether this activity would have involved the participation of partners, especially the Americans. Certainly the need to evacuate South Korean soldiers coming down with malaria reinforces the scarcity of field hospitals capable of handling such patients. At the same time, the point here is not to critique the standards of South Korean biological capabilities but rather to recognize the value of the Vietnam context as an experimental setting in which to encounter diverse field conditions, along with the need to learn and incorporate new forms of treatment. There is a link here to the antiparasite campaigns, moreover, both in the form of the small group of leading researchers (including Dr. Seo), who grew interested in treating new forms of disease in the field, and in the perfection of his craft, handling a difficult task of analysis. Even as malaria remains distinct from the types of parasites typically encountered in South Korea, it provided an opportunity for Dr. Seo to acquire new skills in a related area of research.

This rapid learning curve would soon prove valuable as Dr. Seo and his team published a related study late that same year, this time focusing on intestinal parasites, drawing on two national contexts (South Korea, Vietnam) in examining samples taken from three distinct groups: Vietnamese villagers, U.S. forces stationed in Vietnam, and Koreans, with this last group including troops serving in Vietnam and a control group of forces based at home.[42] Although the diversity sought in the study was motivated by the need for controls, at least nominally, this study, like the previous one, contained a strong element of interest in the more immediate comparison between Korean village life and that of the Vietnamese. Of the four groups, the Koreans led in possessing the highest overall rate for infection, achieving a figure of more than 80 percent and also holding the highest figure for the incidence of polyparasitism, simultaneous infection with more than one type of parasite. If these numbers represented a cause for concern, it was not in the abstract but in the context of the contrast with the Vietnamese, who took an intermediate position between that of the U.S. troops and the Koreans in terms of rates of infection.

If this last point offered little consolation in that Vietnamese villagers experienced fewer infestations on average than did Korean troops, an interesting anomaly in the data offered room for considerable discussion. For reasons that are unclear, Korean troops in Vietnam generally suffered from fewer parasites than did their counterparts based at home, offering an opportunity to explore the possibility of remediation in the near future. Specifically, this point was made with reference to *Ascaris lumbricoides*, among the most common of the parasites in Korea, meaning that something appeared to be happening during the time spent in Vietnam.[43] At the time, Korean forces were not yet receiving anthelminthics, compounds designed specifically to eradicate these pests, so this possibility was eliminated from the outset. Speculation therefore focused on the lifespan of the parasite, with the possibility that prolonged time away from Korea, without any reintroduction of the pest into one's system, might be sufficient to reduce the problem significantly. And as the difference was fairly large—with only slightly more than 15 percent of the forces in Vietnam encountering the problem, as opposed to more than half in Korea—this was a phenomenon requiring further exploration.

Even with the prospect of change, the study offered a sobering portrait of the relative state of health of Korean forces, with a diversity of parasites found in the samples taken. In all, ten different species of helminth ova (the eggs of parasitic worms) and five different species of protozoa showed up, with Korean forces possessing by far the highest rate of infection, both in terms of the overall rate and also in terms of multiple parasites derived from a single source. Finally, the parasites found were not specific to Vietnam, which is to say that many of the same species could be located in both Korea and the battlefield area. Instead of acquiring "exotic" bugs as they relocated to Vietnam, the presumptive claim prior to the study, Korean troops were most likely carrying with them sources of infestation acquired back home. This point is critical in that it contradicts the bias implicit to much of tropical medicine, the notion that certain diseases are endemic only to particular geographical areas and, by extension, can be attributed to certain groups of people. Contrary to expectations, the arriving Koreans found the Vietnamese to be much healthier than their own troops, despite the modesty of their dwellings and the economic circumstances.

As a baseline effort conducted almost simultaneously with start-up of the domestic campaign, these two studies proved enormously valuable in clearing up any misconceptions about the extent of the parasite problem. The second of these, the parasite research in particular, undercut any hopes that the problem could be addressed through a simple comparison with either Vietnamese villagers or American troops, two groups sharing the same space and living conditions throughout the period under study (from 1966 through 1968). With the prevalence of intestinal parasites documented beyond dispute, the challenge now lay in addressing the issue through an aggressive campaign of medical treatment, which took the form of the distribution of anthelminthics, pharmaceuticals capable of killing the pests. As the campaign's lead figures grew increasingly skilled at the collection and analysis of samples, along with the identification of parasites by employing a variety of techniques, they could turn to the problem of acquiring and distributing the necessary remedies in large quantities.

As with family planning in the previous chapter, the need for mass quantities of pharmaceuticals underscored a key shortage in South Korea, that is, the relatively small output of its domestic manufacturers. This is not to say the same thing of the market for such goods; given the ongoing popularity of traditional practice (TKM), it is clear that many Koreans continued to self-medicate in consultation with their visits to practitioners and pharmacies. In contrast, the antiparasite campaigns required a reliable supply of industrially produced medications, available in mass quantities, to be distributed primarily to the nation's schoolchildren following the initial survey of their samples. This set of requirements necessitated an approach of a different magnitude, with the participation of international partners. The campaign also required the cooperation and support of a large population of willing subjects, who had to adapt their behavior to the regimen of taking these new medications regularly and allowing follow-up inspections to establish whether in fact the methods would prove effective.

In this sense, even the compliance demonstrated at the national level through the willing submission of samples in schools was not sufficient to support the broader ambitions of the antiparasite campaign, requiring a renewed effort to reach out to all elements of society. KAPE spread its message through a series of new publications, including *Kŏn'gang* (*Health*), and its associated newsletter *Kŏn'gang sosik* (*Health News*), with these items appearing concurrently with the gearing up for national mobilization in the early 1970s (in 1973 and 1977). The energy and publicity associated with the revised notion of "health" here is fascinating, assigning responsibility for daily maintenance to the individual, much as the family planning campaigns sought to normalize the daily use of reproductive technologies. KAPE much later changed its name to the KAHP (Korean Association for Health Promotion) as the parasite problem began to wane in the late 1980s and early 1990s, but the association and linkage here between these two distinct lexical items—"parasite" and "health"—underscores the centrality of this program to much of South Korean life during the early 1970s.

Mobilizing "Health" (1969 through Late 1978): Distributing Anthelminthics

The incremental "medicalization" of health in South Korea, a process that we have been tracking throughout these chapters, should not imply that the newer publications emerging under the auspices of KAPE would be devoted exclusively to the issue of parasite control. Even a brief survey of a magazine such as *Kŏn'gang* (*Health*), with its first issue appearing in August 1973, indicates that this was not the case. Instead, this magazine and its companion publications, such as *Kŏn'gang sosik* (*Health News*, appearing from 1977), would take a broad approach toward their subject matter, encouraging a spirit of inquiry and promising in return greater confidence, a much higher degree of certainty and control over one's body and life. If this aim could be achieved in part through pharmaceutical means, the pitch was not necessarily framed as a hard sell so much as an appeal to a radically different type of lifestyle. In other words, *Kŏn'gang* had less to do with constructing a singular identification between a person's overall health and the absence of parasites, as admirable a goal as that might have been, and much more to do with instilling a level of confidence in the products of the domestic and international pharmaceutical communities, including an entire range of items bearing little or no direct relation to the antiparasite campaigns. These would include, for example, mild forms of antianxiety medication (meprobamate) and related stronger remedies, even psychotropics (chlorpromazine), although the advertisements for these last two do not specify the conditions under which such a powerful drug might be prescribed.

Moreover, this type of information, now readily available in a doctor's office through a consultation or at a community health center, was aimed not just at promoting a specific type of medication but instead at altering related behavioral and consumption patterns, a much more ambitious goal. To invoke legacy of the family planning campaigns, the distribution of birth control technologies was accompanied with a heavy dose of pedagogy, whether concerning the proper method for insertion of the loop or the designated interval at which to take a birth control pill. Most Koreans were already familiar with ingesting plants and herbal remedies, in other words, but the level of specificity required with pharmaceuticals—measuring the amount of a single dose, as well as regulating the timing between doses—needed to be taught carefully. Starting with the nation's public schools, the antiparasite campaigns therefore constituted an extended case study in teaching familiarization and the use of modern pharmaceuticals on a regular basis, with a nationwide chemotherapy program linked to the initial decade of parasite surveys (1969–1978), aimed at dramatically reducing the rate of infestation.

While officially the rate of compliance was extremely high, as noted previously, there remain numerous apocryphal stories from this period (the early 1970s) concerning the possibility of resistance to the campaigns, employing a variety of methods to evade the scrutiny of the state. Even KAHP acknowledges the reality of such claims and, while not citing a specific figure, recognizes that the campaigns never fully achieved the desired degree of distribution. These methods included passive forms of resistance, for example, students who did not attend school or were absent on a regular basis, as well as more active forms, those who attempted to substitute a sample derived from an animal or an object composed of other organic materials. This type of story, while extremely difficult to pin down with certainty, underscores simultaneously the dark humor and the tension associated with the campaigns, through which the nation sought access to the bodies of its students. In addition to the issue of access, the campaigns brought with them new markers of social distinction, recognizing class and regional differences and reinscribing them in terms of medical categories.

Antiparasite and Mass Chemotherapy: Calibrating the Use of Anthelminthics

These distinctions were to a great extent an unintended consequence of the mass chemotherapy campaigns conducted in conjunction with the antiparasite campaigns, with all students receiving some form of anthelminthic (a parasite-killing compound) at the early stages. This was not the first time that such differences were noted, of course, with health campaigns dating to the colonial period creating a map of the relative distribution and incidence of disease on the peninsula. The argument here is that this was a newer type of distinction enforced by the ROK state, with the presence or absence of parasites serving to mark distinct regional and economic differences. Earlier studies in South Korea had frequently used Cheju Island as a site for limited public health studies, especially for its warm climate and its clear, well-defined boundaries, making for a relatively easy set of control protocols.[44] This convention proved to be more of a convenience than a strict construction of social barriers, although Cheju islanders as a category do make frequent appearances in the South Korean medical literature (from 1948 through the early to mid-1960s) as a form of convenience.

Along with the point concerning the emphasis on social difference, it is critical to recall the visceral, material realities of the antiparasite campaigns, as the majority of accounts have been written as success narratives, framed from the perspective of the present day, when rates of infection tend to remain extremely low. In fact, the start of mass chemotherapy began without a single method or approach taking precedence, meaning that the campaigns constituted, in effect, a comprehensive social experiment. A number of different chemical treatments were used over the course of the succeeding two to three decades, with the ultimate goal aiming toward a cheap, effective solution that could be synthesized domestically and distributed either free or at an extremely low cost. This ambition ran into the problem cited earlier, the issue of patent control, and KAHP openly acknowledges that the South Korean program was willing to violate patent protection in cases where it thought that its public health needs dictated such an action. In effect, KAPE invoked the rhetoric of crisis, using this logic to circumvent any legal or ethical concerns.

In referring earlier to visceral realities, no pun was intended, as the meaning is quite literal. If the campaigns required a dramatic change in behavior, requiring subjects to ingest anthelminthics at specific intervals, it also brought with it a wide range of unpleasant gastrointestinal effects, with a successful use of a drug causing the individual to expel a number of worms and parasite ova from his or her system, typically within a day or two of taking the compound.[45] The rapidity of this cycle was regarded as positive, especially in those cases calling for the repeated administration of drugs in the same community, where a single dose represented only the beginning of an intervention. The life cycle of the parasite in question, the general health of the subject population, and related factors each received consideration in weighing the frequency with which a compound could be distributed to the subjects, especially children and the elderly.

This just goes to say that the South Korean campaign, gearing up for an aggressive response in the early 1970s, had to rely on international models and approaches—while continuing to rely heavily on the Japanese literature—in determining the most effective solution for its *Ascaris* problem. At least initially, the preferred compound was santonin-kainic acid, available through a Japanese manufacturer in pill form. Dosage varied according to age, with the youngest children receiving a single tablet and those over the age of thirteen receiving five tablets. The success narrative generally elides these messy details of calibration, the work of more than two decades (from 1969 through the late 1980s) of fine-tuning and experimentation on a willing subject population. Certainly the effects of the compound on the stomach and intestines could not have been pleasant, nor was the experience of expelling worms from one's system something that could be easily forgotten. At the same time, this was defined as an act of consent, something that individuals did voluntarily.

The extent to which the various subject groups were compliant remains an issue to be explored, moreover, as both schoolchildren and military conscripts have to be addressed as members of a "captive" population, giving their consent, certainly, but perhaps under compromised circumstances. The emergence of newer forms of regulation, such as the IRB (institutional review board), a development dating to the 1960s in the American context, would not take place until much later in South Korea (circa 2006), created only with a perceived need to meet existing international standards. In effect, the program's directors had little oversight other than their own good judgment, and they sometimes included groups of "mentally feeble children" among their test subjects, as this was another population readily available. While we learn little of this last group in terms of their particulars, they make an appearance in at least some of the tests for the effects of anthelminthics, and it is fair to assume they were useful as a typical group of children modeling the effects on the digestive system.

With this emphasis on the material details should come recognition that the pharmaceutical regimen to be employed as part of mass chemotherapy was rarely tied to a single item and that, much like the case with family planning, this next series of steps involved a good deal of tinkering over the course of two to three decades. The initial use of compounds such as santonin-kainic acid (from 1969 through the early 1970s), along with piperazine (from 1971 to 1981), tended to reflect accessible sources or supplies from nearby suppliers, most frequently Japanese pharmaceutical manufacturers. These methods were later supplemented by pyrantel pamoate (from 1973 through 1988) before giving way in succession to more effective compounds, including mebendazole (from 1983 to 1993) and albendazole (from 1988 to 1995), with these last two produced in the ROK as a result of refinements to domestic manufacture.[46] Again, the loose analogy to a clinical trial remains appropriate here, as the KAPE was not only seeking to eliminate the parasites but, more important, to determine the most cost-effective means of doing so.

While the government was making adjustments to the chemical regimen, the experience of participating remained fairly uniform, at least for the first several cycles. Twice yearly, following the sampling procedure, students received a dose of the prevailing form of treatment, typically administered in oral form. This did leave room for evasion, at least through the possibility of not swallowing the medication, but the school could record its figures and still assume a relatively high rate of compliance. As outlined here, the days immediately following ingestion of the medication were likely uncomfortable, with mild to severe gastrointestinal distress, and with material expelled from the body in the form of deceased worms and their ova. As uncomfortable as this was, this was a common experience, shared by students of a particular school with members of their age cohort. As long as infection rates remained high, the government promoted mass chemotherapy as its approach, with this policy changing only when progress had been achieved.

At this early stage, the KAPE regarded geography primarily from the standpoint of rates of compliance, focusing on those areas likely to hold out or to present problems in terms of taking samples. Not surprisingly, there was a correlation between the distance from one of the three major metropoles (Seoul, Pusan, and Daegu) and the likelihood of having a significant number of individuals who had yet to submit their samples. More specifically, this meant the northeast area of Kangwŏn-do, as well as a large section of the southwest, the latter traditionally perceived as a poorer agricultural area. As the program grew in emphasis, it is clear that the problems associated with these two areas began to assume the character of a distinct impression, although how rigid this characterization became remains subject to debate. Certainly the shift from mass chemotherapy to selected medication revealed those areas where the parasite problem persisted, with this bringing a range of negative associations.[47]

In making this observation, I do not want to offer a simple comparison between the legacy of Japanese colonial practice and that of these more recent public health campaigns by the postcolonial state. Rather, my intent is to illustrate the multiple, strange, and fascinating ways in which the Park state—along with subsequent South Korean governments—echoed and remade Japanese precedents. If the effects of the antiparasite campaigns were ultimately less pernicious because they reflected nationalist aims, the economic and social divide between those regions that achieved "success" and those that failed cannot and should not be ignored. At the level of the individual, moreover, the transition from mass chemotherapy to selected targeting, taking aside those children with parasitic worms, also tended to reinforce these social divisions, particularly as South Korea started to become a more affluent society. Certainly by the early to mid- to late 1980s, schoolchildren would have been aware of their peers who were asked to stay after class, aware that something was amiss.

With time providing a good deal of perspective, the early stages of the mass chemotherapy effort approximated a nationwide clinical trial, something not easily replicated in today's South Korea. To review, the Park state was able to mobilize nationally on two major fronts, appealing to nationalism in terms of the health of its South Korean soldiers fighting abroad, while simultaneously emphasizing the domestic context. The almost complete absence of civil society meant that there were few questions raised about the methods of sample gathering and, more important, about the mass distribution of chemical remedies that were still very much in development. By later in the program, the most effective methods were mobilized with far more certainty, meaning that the remaining demographic suffering from infection could be treated in a timely manner. What this elides, however, is a deep, visceral history in which the donation of a sample became an uncomfortable and necessary reality, as was its aftermath, typically involving the ingestion of a new drug and the accompanying expulsion of worms from one's intestines over the following period of two to three days.

Refashioning Parasites and Health: Legacies?

Along with the key image opening this chapter, a young boy defending his rice from the unwanted attentions of a giant *Ascaris*, a related image serves to provide a framing context for its closure, that of a second poster which appeared regularly in *Health News* in the late 1970s. Asking viewers to attend to the inspection ritual twice annually, the image of a large microscope associated the act of consent with national fitness ("national strength"), connoting physical fitness specifically but also implying national integrity, with its attending economic and commercial implications. By this point, late in the rule of Park Chung Hee, the first national survey data were just coming in, attesting to the "success" of the program, at least as framed by the criteria of reducing rates of infection. Even as South Korea had ended its presence in Vietnam, the nation maintained its military conscription policy, with a need to keep soldiers in the best possible condition.

For its part, KAPE did not change its name to KAHP until 1986, indicating the waning of the parasite as the sole or singular target of the organization, with a corresponding shift in emphasis to a broader set of health initiatives. Strictly speaking, KAHP existed as early as 1982 in some form, with formal merger of the two bodies then taking place at the later date. Over a period of slightly more than two decades, KAHP (1964 to 1986) conducted the work of going into the nation's schools, collecting samples, and distributing a range of anthelminthic measures on the return portion of the cycle. As with family planning in the preceding chapter, this legacy should not only evoke older associations dating to the prewar era but also the comparative context of its immediate neighbors, as South Korea sought to distinguish itself from many of these same nations.

And the very tool that had made this work possible, parasitology, also took a revised form within the Korean academy. With the waning of the parasite issue as a domestic problem by the early 1990s, programs such as the one at Seoul National University had to adopt new targets, in this case placing the focus almost exclusively on the external. For SNU, parasitology gave way to a focus on tropical medicine, with the nation using its acquired expertise to target its neighbors and partners. With South Korea today experiencing a renewal of its close relationship with Southeast Asia—including Vietnam, the Philippines, and Myanmar, among others—it should come as no surprise that Korean tropical medicine has the potential to act as a form of soft power and diplomacy, this time on behalf of a "developed" nation reaching out to share its own models of expertise.

6 Reconstructing the Face: "Asian Blepharoplasty," Professional Expertise, and the Development of a Plastic Surgery Market, 1954 to the Present

"A Plastic Surgeon's Paradise" (1953–1954): Making Transformative Claims through Surgery

"American Goodwill in Asia"

In late 1953, Dr. David Ralph Millard (1919–2011) was commissioned as part of a U.S. Marine Corps surgical team to remain behind in South Korea to continue the work of providing humanitarian relief, or, as he would characterize his task, one of offering "visible evidence of American goodwill in Asia."[1] Specifically, Dr. Millard served as a plastic surgeon for the Marine Corps (1954–1955), performing a wide variety of reconstructive procedures, including skin grafts and the repair of the cleft lip; for the latter of these he later became best known.[2] A 1944 graduate of Harvard Medical School, Millard had already accumulated significant clinical experience prior to his enlistment, having trained first as a resident (between 1948 and 1949) in the United Kingdom with Dr. Harold D. Gillies (1882–1960), with whom he would coauthor the two-volume set, *The Principles and Art of Plastic Surgery* (1957), before serving additional time (from 1949 to 1952) at several locations in the United States.[3] By the time he had arrived in South Korea in November 1953, Millard had extensive knowledge of the most recent surgical techniques associated with a variety of congenital defects, but this would be his first encounter with the immediate exigencies of war and its aftermath.[4]

Millard's mentor and predecessor, Harold Gillies, had pioneered many of the experimental techniques associated with the nascent field of plastic surgery, making his reputation by repairing the faces of British soldiers injured during World War I. From his base at Queen Mary's Hospital (1917), Gilles would attempt to minimize damage inflicted by war, typically caused by gunshot wounds, using a series of skin grafts to cover visible signs of wounds or scars. As the damage was sometimes quite extensive, Gilles confronted the problem of keeping skin tissue alive, learning how to relocate it from one part of the body to another by crafting a series of grafts, or flaps of skin, known as pedicles. Nearly four decades later, Millard traveled to a very different part of the world, but his challenge remained similar in many respects: that of treating both civilian and military injuries and arriving in the immediate aftermath of a brutal civil war that had witnessed new means of injuring the human body, especially the face.

Drafted primarily as a replacement for doctors who had completed their surgical rotations through South Korea, Millard has since acknowledged his reluctance to travel, uncertain of the value of his work in this new context, whether to the Marines or to members of the South Korean population, who had expressed reluctance at making use of American facilities. Soon, though, he discovered that the combination of the recent Korean War and a legacy of neglect would provide ample opportunities for his brand of intervention, with surgical procedures carried out under local anesthesia and with skin grafts and pedicle flaps serving as an improvised solution to repair any number of defects.[5] Along with other American doctors present at that time, Millard came to recognize the unusual opportunity he had been given for rapid professional development because of the sheer diversity of cases that he would encounter. The orphanages associated with refugee populations rapidly became a popular site to search for potential patients, along with Korean leper colonies, which he went so far as to describe as "a lifetime of reconstruction."[6] Only several months into his tenure, Millard enthused that "this [Korea] was indeed a plastic surgeon's paradise."[7]

Although he put his skills to use in a range of clinical situations, Millard quickly became fascinated with the difficult task of facial reconstruction, especially for those patients who had experienced severe burn damage during the recent Korean conflict.[8] In his estimation, many of these cases could be best approached through the creation of eyebrow flaps: "To give eyebrows to this face [a burn victim] helps to relieve the monotony for they serve as twin oasis [sic] in a desert of skin grafts."[9] This type of work would motivate Millard to think further about the identity of his South Korean patients; he did similar work with American military patients, including both white and black soldiers, as Korea was the first war in which integrated American units would serve.[10] In his account, these circumstances next led Millard to contemplate the type of surgery for which he would receive a great deal of notoriety, particularly among scholars of Asian American studies, who frequently cite his work as a typical example of (American) medical excess in an overseas setting.[11] This is because Millard began to focus on the eye socket, the eyelids, and the folds of skin situated in the surrounding tissue, especially in terms of creating new perceptions concerning a patient's ethnic identity.

The critical transition came with his realization that existing work with the Z plasty—the technique of working with tiny, triangular folds of skin, approximating a Z shape, typically to camouflage or minimize the visibility of a scar—could also be used to create a very different style of visage. According to Millard's account, a Korean translator working with U.S. forces came to him requesting to be "made into a round-eye."[12] Uncertain of how to proceed, Millard determined that "the flat nose and the oriental eye were the two features which seemed to lend themselves to the most striking change with the least radical form of intervention."[13] The two features could be altered in conjunction, in other words, with a change to the nose cartilage producing a corresponding effect on the prominence of the epicanthic fold of the neighboring eye. Altering the bridge of the nose alone could not accomplish the project as envisioned, but Millard claimed that he began to receive similar requests from other Korean patients requesting a comparable version of the same procedure, that is, a cartilage transplant to the nasal bridge. This first step, along with subsequent work performed on the epicanthic fold itself, completed the process of producing a "round eye," with removal of the fold along with any excess skin around the upper eyelid area.

While we never learn the interpreter's response to his surgery, Millard implies a satisfied patient, noting the man's subsequent conversion to Christianity, along with his plans to travel to the United States to study for the ministry.[14] Moreover, the transformation of his identity is complete in this version (B), with Millard commenting that many viewers now took the man "for Mexican or Italian" following the surgery.[15] By labeling this section of his publication "Oriental to Occidental," Millard makes explicit the assumption that he was helping his patients to establish a complete transformation of their identity and, moreover, one that accomplished a desired aim for members of this self-selecting population. It is precisely the ease and confidence with which he characterizes this problematic series of gestures that has since earned Millard a great deal of commentary from scholars of ethnicity and Asian American studies.[16] My goal here consists of neither criticizing Millard's motives nor defending his surgical procedure's legacy but rather of historicizing this type of surgical work within the broader context of the intense encounter between the worlds of South Korean and American military medicine both during and following the Korean War, especially as this type of procedure was gradually reintroduced into South Korean society in recent decades.

The transition from previous medical models—with "Korean" medicine, here defined broadly as a complex hybrid, encompassing several distinct traditions, including Chinese, Japanese (German academic medicine), and the various international relief efforts associated with the Korean War—has been a dominant theme throughout these chapters, but it is particularly important here as we begin to consider the development of new possibilities for reconstructive work in the mid-1950s. If these concerns required several decades of legal, medical, and institutional change before South Koreans embraced this type of procedure in the form of their own reconfigured medical institutions, Millard's intervention nonetheless places the related questions of personal appearance, identity, and self-perception at the center of the encounter with American military medicine. More critical than the surgery itself as a procedure was the postwar context in which it took place, with medical relief frequently mobilized as evidence of benevolent intentions, conveniently ignoring the conspicuous power differences embedded within the U.S.–ROK relationship.

This encounter is precisely where Millard hoped to situate his work, after all, as his interest lay with improving medical care and surgical techniques, and he was conscious of the American military presence not just in South Korea but also distributed throughout much of Northeast Asia. He made no attempt to claim priority for his surgery and, in fact, recognized that many other variations of the procedure existed in the region.[17] For South Korea, the effort to reshape the area around the eye generally consisted of the removal of a narrow strip of skin from the upper eyelid, producing a "temporary ectropion" (a type of protrusion or bulge), causing the lower eyelid to turn outward.[18] With the reduction of swelling following surgery, the practice generally produced an eye shape closer to the desired double fold, even as Millard found such an approach lacking. His account goes on to locate this example in the context of his experiences of the region's military hospitals, including

Tokyo and Hong Kong, reinforcing a comparative baseline, constructing a context around his work by setting it within a larger network of related developments. The question remains, however, as to the problematic character of his claim to be able to render a complete transformation of a patient's identity.

Distinguishing "Reconstructive" Work and the "Aesthetic"

If we defer these intersecting issues of surgical priority and identity construction until a later point, Millard's work serves as a valuable marker of the complex relationship between the immediate context of the war and the heightening of emerging concerns around personal identity. Before closing his article, he reminds his audience that this kind of surgical phenomenon will likely not be confined to Northeast Asia, as there "have been well over 10,000 Japanese war brides as well as many post-war marriages with Korean girls."[19] To translate these issues into a more recent vocabulary, Millard understood that his surgical practice might have transnational implications, with the "new" faces moving along with the bodies of his (presumably) satisfied clients. This point raises the related issue of the distinction between reconstructive surgery and its more recent counterpart, aesthetic or plastic surgery (*sŏnghyŏng oekwa*), with the former category constituting a significant number of surgeries in the South Korean setting at about this same time. Both soldiers and civilians had suffered a great deal from loss of limbs and severe injuries, and, as with Millard's service in the Marines, many other doctors found an opportunity to promote their interests while simultaneously conveying the benevolent intentions of the American people.

Of the many figures to be associated with this style of post–Korean War relief work, Dr. Howard A. Rusk (1901–1989) is perhaps the most prominent, best known in the United States as a pioneer of rehabilitative medicine, especially at the Rusk Institute of Rehabilitation Medicine, based at New York University, which he helped to found in the late 1940s.[20] Starting his work with the care of injured airmen during World War II, Dr. Rusk began to expand the range of his patient base in the postwar period, including a group of disabled miners, a population in which he became interested due to a developing relationship with John L. Lewis and the United Mine Workers Welfare Fund.[21] Before the outbreak of the Korean War, Rusk was already a significant figure in the worlds of medicine and fund raising, which made him an ideal candidate when his next opportunity came along. In Rusk's account, his awareness of Korea did not extend much beyond newspaper headlines until early 1953, at which point he was invited as part of a visiting team to investigate the health problems associated with the ongoing conflict.[22]

Prior to this visit, Korea had served primarily as a hindrance to Rusk, as his efforts to secure federal dollars for his ambitious plans for the rehabilitation of veterans were generally met with concerns about the federal budget crisis.[23] His host during the visit, the American-Korean Foundation (AKF), had been founded in 1952 with the intent of mobilizing funds and supplies for the relief of Korean refugees affected by the war, and the invitation to tour Korea was part of a strategy to bring in prominent Americans like Dr. Rusk to aid the project.[24] Along with treating the more conspicuous signs of illness—prominent among these were tuberculosis and leprosy—Rusk almost immediately recognized the powerful conflux of interests between his project in rehabilitative medicine and the Korean context.[25] Rather than seeking federal aid, he soon became a powerful advocate on behalf of the AKF, assuming presidency of the organization in 1954, while continuing to regard these two projects, rehabilitative medicine and the Korea setting, as mutually beneficial in terms of increasing potential sources of revenue and raising public awareness about his mission.

In brief, Rusk's project and the AKF made for a reciprocal arrangement, as the doctor lent his considerable expertise in fund raising and public relations to channel much-needed resources to the group. In turn, the AKF would provide Rusk with a platform—and a steady supply of Korean bodies as subjects—on which to mobilize his larger concerns about rehabilitative medicine, expanding his New York base to include a growing set of national and international partners.[26] Not surprisingly, the initial report issued in conjunction with the "Rusk Mission to Korea" focused on portraying the Korean conflict in the starkest terms possible, capturing the broad strokes of the war in a manner likely to elicit the sympathy of potential donors. As the opening paragraph put it succinctly, "Four years of fighting have resulted in nearly 1,000,000 civilian casualties and the complete destruction of 500,000 homes, 9,000,000 dislocated people, 100,000 orphans, 300,000 war widows, and 15, 000 amputees."[27] Milton Eisenhower (1899–1985), brother to the U.S. president and head of Penn State University from 1950 through 1956, assumed the role of chairman of the AKF, underscoring the growing cultural significance attributed to the group, despite its nominal character as a voluntary organization.

For our concern here, the Rusk mission, along with its associated work through the AKF, would be absolutely critical in promoting the increasing "traffic" in bodies, ideas, and medical practices traveling between South Korea and the United States. Initially, this consisted primarily of Korean trainees traveling to the United States for study tours, that is, doctors and student nurses funded by new scholarship sources.[28] This represented only a portion of the exchange, however, and the more interesting part lies within the broad category of ideas and practices: If Dr. Rusk continued to focus his efforts in Manhattan, finding new ways to improve the lives of wounded soldiers, many of his ideas and new techniques soon made it to Korea in some form through a variety of AKF-funded projects. Physical therapy, occupational therapy, and the project of rehabilitation began to reach Korean children as early as the mid-1950s, for example, especially through the National Rehabilitation Center at Tongnae (Pusan), with new recreation and child development programs playing a major part.[29] While there were many more patients than the AKF could possibly accommodate, the point here remains valid; namely, that individuals injured during the war were exposed to a variety of postsurgical options in the form of new therapies and the possibility of receiving replacement limbs.

If we place the shared concerns of Drs. Millard and Rusk in the mid-1950s side by side, the distinction between the two types of surgery become less clear, certainly in terms of a common set of motives informing a desire to restore the body and spirit of the wounded veteran or civilian. Even as some of Dr. Millard's clients requested a change in appearance, his work in Korea derived primarily from the context of war, again, dealing primarily with the victims of burn damage. In these cases, the surgeries performed on the face, while aesthetic in a limited sense, were informed equally by a project of restoring a sense of identity to the victim, constituting a project of reconstruction. And if the Korean War context does not necessarily represent the first case of such surgery in South Korea, it nonetheless represents a point of departure for much of the subsequent surgical practice in the nation, with South Korean surgeons dramatically transforming their practice during the course of their interactions with American and international colleagues.[30] The critical question lies in exploring how these forms of practice would be transformed over the next several decades (from the early 1960s through the mid-1990s) to the point where "Asian blepharoplasty," or surgery on the eyelids (*ssangkkŏp'ul*), would become a very different type of practice, one of the most commonly requested procedures among both South Korean men and women.[31]

The intermediate stages required to execute such a transition were multiple, and this chapter will focus primarily on the accompanying medical, legal, and institutional changes that brought about an aggressively commercial South Korean medical practice by the late 1980s and early 1990s, following professionalization and legal recognition. Reading Millard's work, along with that of Dr. Rusk, as simply an American intervention adopted wholesale by Koreans would be far too facile an approach, and while I sympathize with many of the criticisms of Millard, what I aim for here is a lengthy process of cultural negotiation and technical exchange, whereby South Korean surgeons remade their surgical practice from a diverse set of elements borrowed from abroad as well as those deriving from domestic and regional sources. South Korean health care has long maintained a progressive narrative—one largely unsupported by its history—and the core of this story lies in a set of ideological markers that continue to carry over from the Korean War's aftermath, when the nation was the recipient of multilateral sources of aid. Both Millard and Rusk based their projects in this period, when medical relief work carried with it very specific humanitarian and, by extension, anticommunist themes.

As previously mentioned, AKF maintained a very high profile through at least the second half of the 1950s, with its connection to Milton Eisenhower making relationships possible with any of a number of prominent political and fund-raising figures, including members of the Rockefeller family. Brochures for the foundation sought to reach as wide an audience as possible, sponsoring an ambitious array of aid projects—collected under the rubric of "Health, Education, Welfare"—designed to reach directly to the lives of Korean "orphans, war widows, students, nurses, [and] teachers."[32] If these materials were largely designed for an American audience, the means through which the aid was conveyed on the Korean end nonetheless reinforced the notion that a great deal of medical assistance derived from abroad, even if the ideological content was likely not as accessible to the recipients. As in Chapter 3, with the discussion of the Minnesota Project, Korean doctors and nurses training at this time would have experienced a rare opportunity to study abroad in a limited number of cases and, in many others, to work alongside their international colleagues in newly refurbished hospitals and clinics.

It is these types of settings that we need to consider as we trace the origins and growth of a South Korean plastic surgery community from its modest beginnings in the early 1960s at Yonsei University and a handful of similar sites to its flourishing state today, with the latter development most closely linked to the rise of private clinics in southeastern Seoul, the area south of the Han River. The context of reconstructive surgery introduced by Dr. Rusk in 1953, with its emphasis on the body, typically involving a major injury or loss of a limb, suggests a specialty populated most frequently by orthopedic surgeons. If the work performed by Dr. Millard does not necessarily fall under the broad category of maxillofacial surgery, that is, reconstruction of the head, neck, jaws, and face, his impulse nonetheless led him to portray much of the work as motivated by a similar set of concerns. The critical question to approach then is how the practice of South Korean surgeons has migrated from this early ideological and reconstructive context in the post–Korean War period to one in which external appearance matters above all else, promoting surgery primarily as a personal choice based on economic motives. More important, how and why have South Korean patients come to embrace this culture, earning for the nation the recent nickname of "the Republic of Plastic Surgery"?

Crafting a "Korean" Surgical Practice: Reconstruction to Professionalization (1955–1974)

Surgical Precedents: From "Oriental" to "Asian" Blepharoplasty

If the more recent usage of the category "Asian" blepharoplasty will be treated as the dominant form of eye surgery, it may come as something of a surprise to recognize that numerous variants of the term were already in use in the mid-twentieth century, particularly as competing varieties of the eye surgery spread throughout the region. The general category of "Oriental" served as a convenient mid-century rubric with which to capture the diverse forms of plastic surgery being performed in a range of locations, including the Philippines, Singapore, Korea, Japan, and Hawaii, with this ethnic label often used to refer to the eye surgery procedure.[33] With the earliest published accounts dating to nineteenth-century Japan, the surgery itself was by no means new when Millard first began to popularize it in the mid-1950s. What was new was the perception of a measure of self-transformation afforded by the procedure and, perhaps more important, the added sense of control that accompanied these changes. While we will not focus on the perceptions of patients here, the surgery also offered the possibility of community to a set of South Korean doctors, who could mobilize their practice around it (and related procedures) to achieve a specific set of professional aspirations.

The goal of professionalization required nearly two decades to achieve (1955–1974), however, as the immediate post–Korean War period did not permit much space for aesthetic concerns and related forms of bodily enhancement. Instead, much of the attention devoted to the body for this period tended to focus almost exclusively on reconstructive work, and this would remain true for someone like Dr. Millard, who was far better known for his work with the palate, repairing congenital defects to the lips and the roof of the mouth.[34] The face as an object of concern would receive attention in terms of repairing damage—whether inflicted by the war or congenital—to allow an individual to function more comfortably within society. The ideological message conveyed through much of this work, providing humanitarian aid at a peak in the early Cold War, would place the faces of South Korean children and patients conspicuously on posters and publicity materials, creating a perception of need that lingers to the present.[35] But this does not address the critical issue of how these individuals saw themselves nor that of the means by which a domestic medical community would begin to develop its own sets of skills and expertise.

To reiterate a point made with the introduction of Millard's work, South Korean surgeons were coming to the procedure not as something entirely new but as a form of practice situated within a diverse pool of resources. Drawing on an extensive body of literature within the East Asian context, with Japanese (and Chinese) published sources dating to the late nineteenth century, South Korean doctors had the choice of selecting from among multiple options. Among these materials, the most commonly cited include the work of Mikamo (1896), Uchida (1926), and Maruo (1929), with the common element to these early accounts lying in the use of sutures to link the upper eyelid to the tarsal ridge, that is, the tissue situated immediately above the eyebrow.[36] After the removal of these sutures several days later, the appearance would be of a "double eyelid," with a furrow, the palpebral sulcus, now marking a crease where previously there had appeared a single eyelid. These sources, along with a number of similar Meiji- and Taisho-era publications from Japan, offer a fascinating peek into the surgery prior to mid-twentieth century interventions and have sparked a lively debate concerning the possible effects of Westernization on perceptions of beauty within greater East Asia.[37]

The conspicuous anatomical differences between the "Asian" and "Western" face, broadly construed, tend to concentrate on the area of the eyes due to differences in the position and amount of the tissue situated in the area, with approximately half or more of Asian patients typically possessing a common set of features in this region. These features may include an absent or poorly defined superior palpebral fold, the presence of periorbital fat, and an epicanthal fold of varying configuration and size. The classic "double eyelid" surgery of the present day therefore centers on these features, attempting to emphasize the two folds in particular so as to approximate the rough contours of the desired "round eye." While the earliest accounts of eye surgery predate the nineteenth century, accounts from the late nineteenth century mark the first appearance of procedures that center on a concern with the aesthetic specifically, one likely mediated by the increased frequency of contact and trade with Western cultures.

One of the more influential accounts of these developments, Sander Gilman's *Making the Body Beautiful* (1999), briefly considers the Japanese case in a section devoted to "Oriental Noses and Eyes."[38] For Gilman, the periodization for eye surgery retains the broad contours suggested here, beginning with Mikamo, and his evidence lies in two major lines of inquiry: first, the surgical legacy and, next, the record of the visual arts. As for the former, Gilman cites a total of thirty-two different procedures developed in Japan specific to surgery on the eyelid spanning roughly a half-century (from 1896 through 1945), although, curiously, he declines to provide full citations for some of these cases. The latter form of evidence proves more convincing, especially when he appeals to "the ideal form of the face as captured in Japanese traditional portraiture," seeking to capture incremental changes in aesthetic preference.[39] Here, changes to the eyelid are placed within the context of the entire face, and Gilman makes the case for the emergence of a formative ideal in process, one reflecting the increasing influence of Westernization. If his views on the surgery are less extreme than those of Millard, Gilman nonetheless places it within a continuum in which a critical shift has taken place, one favoring a stylized image borrowed from abroad.[40]

To revisit the terms of this debate, Millard's controversial take on the transformation from "Oriental to Occidental" inflates his personal role as the agent of transformation and tends to either elide or minimize the contributions of his many predecessors. The surgery was already well known to doctors throughout the region, with the Japanese medical community publishing most frequently on this subject, an influence that would very likely have reached the South Korean medical community, possibly even in the prewar period.[41] Moreover, even with the influence of the West on Meiji Japan, the identity attached to the surgery was anything but straightforward. In fact, many scholars of the surgery argue that it does not connote "the West" per se but instead marks a form of difference within a broader Asian context, with a double fold underscoring a conception of beauty that remains essentially Asian.[42] In other words, according to this revised account, patients are not trying to alter their ethnic identity in any radical fashion but simply wish to distinguish themselves from their peers by creating a more pleasing appearance. In this revised account, Millard serves more as a popularizer than an innovator per se, and it is from this takeoff point that South Korean surgeons would most likely have begun to develop their own work.

The Migration of Bodies and Practices

Moreover, these first South Korean surgeons had a wider range of options from which to choose beginning in the second half of the 1950s, as the eye surgery was becoming increasingly popular at a number of different sites scattered throughout greater Asia. Although the literature originating from Japan remained the most prominent, B. T. Sayoc, based in the Philippines, began to publish his papers in the following decade in English-language journals, with the earliest of these appearing in Philippine journals as early as 1954.[43] Similarly, Dr. Khoo Boo-Chai of Singapore performed the surgery from about 1959, publishing his results in the early 1960s. For Dr. Khoo, the prevalence of the eye surgery was fascinating in itself, as it constituted nearly two-thirds of the procedures he performed in his practice; and he speculated that this trend held true for other surveys originating within Asia.[44] In terms of practice, the procedure had not changed substantially, with preferred methods including the creation of the palpebral fold, as outlined previously, and a conjunctival approach.[45] In the latter case, the major difference lay in the placement of the stitches on the inner surface of the lower eyelid, thus hiding any possible scarring, whereas previously any marks would have appeared externally, visible on surface of the skin.

With minor variations, these two related clusters of surgical activity, the first appearing in Japan prior to the close of the war (between 1896 and the early 1930s), the second appearing in various parts of Asia following the conflict (from 1945 to 1963), would have represented points of entry for aspiring South Korean surgeons coming to the practice in the late 1950s and early 1960s. The major distinction between the two periods, along with the temporal intervention of the war, had primarily to do with the degree of intervention intended, with this remark including the number of stitches introduced, their placement, and the decision of whether to proceed with additional tissue removal, including the underlying muscle and fat. As the type of surgery became more aggressive, in other words, some physicians began to remove strips of skin from the area above the eyelid, even going so far as to remove muscle and fat tissue from the same location. This gesture would have enhanced the effect of a "round eye" to a greater extent, at least according to the aesthetic conventions of the time.

The spread and popularity of the procedure, with minor variations across the region, may be attributed to postwar economic recovery and the corresponding restoration of a comparable level of health care, one that could include aesthetic concerns along with basic needs. If the issue of "Westernization" remains controversial in terms of determining a patient's aims, most observers credit the Japanese for establishing priority for the surgery, noting a lengthy tradition of modification to the eyelid during the first half of the twentieth century. The postwar arrival of large numbers of outsiders in neighboring locations including the Philippines, Hawaii, Korea, and Singapore then represents the next phase of the cycle, with the popularity of surgery growing rapidly and with an increasingly sophisticated range of techniques available. Millard's attempt to place himself at the head of this second development does not stand up to scrutiny, at least certainly not to the extent that he might claim to be an innovator. In addition, scholars have labeled his rhetorical aim of promoting identity transformation as a distortion, or, at the very least, a "misunderstanding."[46] If South Korean–language publications on blepharoplasty do not appear frequently at this point, economic factors and recovery from the war offer a plausible explanation.

At about the same time, and geographically close to South Korea, the plastic surgery industry in Japan was flourishing again, meaning that its trajectory and the scope of its influence cannot be limited simply to the prewar period. According to the survey, *Venus Envy* (1997), Tokyo became a center for such activity by the early 1960s, roughly a decade removed from the American occupation (1945 through 1952), and then in the midst of what would prove to be a lengthy economic boom.[47] With more than 100 clinics based in the city, and a clientele loosely estimated at over 200,000 per year, the Japanese plastic surgery community served not only a large number of domestic patients, but increasingly women traveling from nearby sites in the region.[48] These clients included a small number of Vietnamese after 1965, with that country also developing its own plastic surgery industry in conjunction with the arrival of a significant American presence. In Haiken's estimation, the critical issue of changing racial and aesthetic ideals rarely emerged explicitly in these settings; instead, the pragmatics of medical practice and achieving a means of reaching a target audience tended to dominate the conversation.

Thailand was also heavily influenced by the war in Southeast Asia, with its military receiving substantial American aid packages as part of a regional infrastructural buildup for the conduct of the war. Many of the B-52 bombers that would take part in "Operation Rolling Thunder," the series of intense bombing campaigns over North Vietnam, departed from and returned to Thai airbases. An unexpected corollary to this increased military activity was an overhaul of the Thai tourism industry, with the corresponding promotion of the sex trade and the related transformation of the medical community. Ara Wilson underscores this point by arguing that "military activity has been integral to advancing Thai medical technologies, including the skills used in elective cosmetic surgery."[49] In simple terms, the identity issues raised by more frequent contact with Westerners, along with increased opportunities for Thai doctors to study abroad, began to transform the practice of surgery, in terms of both its level of expertise and its more widespread availability on a commercial basis. While this point has to remain speculative, it is fair to consider the extent to which South Korea was possibly influenced by regional developments in surgical practice taking place in Japan and Southeast Asia at the beginning of the 1960s.

If the traffic in bodies derived in large part from the surrounding region, there were also limited interactions with North America. Identity issues emerged more openly with the spread of surgeries to Asians living in North America, a development likely dating to the 1920s, before intensifying in the postwar period, especially by the mid-1950s. Many of these stories involve marriage or serious relationships between partners from different ethnic groups, with one of the pair opting for some form of surgery. In one famous case, Shima Kito, a Japanaese male, underwent surgery to his nose and eyelids, ultimately winning the bride of his choice and in the process reinventing himself as "William White."[50] Less extreme than this, some Korean War brides would undergo eye surgery after relocating with their husbands to America, finding that the procedure eased the transition, both for the sake of the relationship and in terms of meeting the expectations of a new community. This last case is particularly useful as we return to South Korea because even the contemporary plastic surgery market exceeds the confines of Seoul and has to include frequent traffic between Seoul and Los Angeles, not to mention that taking place between other common sites of migration.

Professionalization in South Korea (1954–1974)

At the earliest stages (from 1954 through 1960), South Korean professional organizations devoted strictly to plastic (*sŏnghyŏng oekwa*) or aesthetic (*miyong sŏnghyŏng oekwa*) surgery did not formally exist, and practitioners of eye surgery were grouped under traditional anatomical categories or subspecialties, such as ophthalmology. Concern for the face and the area around the eyes centered largely on questions of repairing damage, as the context of reconstructive surgery from the war years continued to dominate through the early 1960s. If there was a small subset of practitioners at this time, culturally their practice appeared superfluous, if not outright indulgent, and patients tended to be regarded as possessing a psychological, rather than physical, set of concerns. To frame this in terms of a different vocabulary, plastic surgery did not yet possess a distinct identity linked to aesthetic purposes—with the community still overlapping primarily with orthopedics—and patients tended to attract negative attention when they received any attention at all.

At the same time, there were many advantages to this gradual approach. With the relatively late development of South Korean surgical practice, practitioners benefited from the postwar growth of new techniques and increasingly sophisticated forms of practice, especially with many of these events taking place in neighboring countries. In the Japanese context, Shirakabe notes the rapid growth of interest in the procedure toward the end of the American occupation, with eight reports of the double eyelid surgery appearing between the years 1950 and 1951, a development he attributes to the wider availability and better regulation of anesthesia used for surgical purposes.[51] If Shirakabe's main goal lies in tying the surgery to a lengthy Japanese lineage, for which he makes a convincing case, he acknowledges the role of international contributors in the postwar period, with Fernandez (1960) chief among these.[52] The removal of underlying skin and muscle tissue, a more radical form of excision in Shirakabe's estimation, underscores a new trend toward a preference for eyes set deeper in the face, indicating that there was not yet a single style or desired aim in terms of achieving a final result.

Collectively, this discussion reinforces the earlier claim that the emergence of a South Korean community of plastic surgeons, with regular publications beginning to appear only in the early to mid-1970s, benefited enormously in terms of improved surgical technique and better materials with which to work.[53] Aesthetic concerns were shaped by the local context, and, as Shirakabe notes, the preferences would change frequently with fashion. For South Korean doctors specifically, this meant not only a substantial market in performing the surgery but also a secondary market in correcting or altering procedures done without achieving a sufficient level of client satisfaction.[54] We will return to these developments later, along with the creation of an export-oriented market for plastic surgery, in the interest of focusing here on the critical question of legal recognition as professionals. Following the official formation of the Korean Society of Plastic and Reconstructive Surgeons (1966), legal and institutional reforms made a more viable form of practice possible, although substantial growth did not take place until at least the mid-1980s, when the economy had reached a level capable of supporting a substantial client base.

Even as coverage for this transitional period remains minimal, there was a small group of recognized practitioners, as illustrated by the formation of a Department of Plastic Surgery and Reconstructive Surgery at Yonsei University as early as 1961, offering instruction to students beginning in 1964.[55] Although the specialty was not yet fully recognized and would not receive official status until early in the next decade, this small group of professionals was interested in building a community and, at the same time, in rigorously policing its boundaries. The practice of paraffin injection, used to augment the breasts, arrived from Japan probably sometime around the late 1960s, and this type of unsanctioned activity gave some physicians an unsavory reputation, making all the more difficult the task of building the field as a reputable one.[56] For all of these reasons—economic, cultural, and ethical—the South Korean field of plastic surgery needed to devote its energy to cultivating allies and strengthening professional ties before it could make any gestures toward cultivating a wider public and clientele.

This process of consolidation occupied much of the late 1960s and early 1970s, culminating in the October 1973 recognition of the field as a new subspecialty within the broader field of medicine.[57] This revision to existing medical law was not designed with plastic surgery alone in mind but rather sought to regulate the growth of numerous subspecialties that had grown up in the intervening period. Between 1966 and 1973, for example, plastic surgeons had successfully lobbied for recognition within the KMA (Korean Medical Association), achieving the desired result in 1969. Formal recognition in the early 1970s now meant that the practice could be regarded as legitimate, and if this did not radically change the material practice of surgery itself—there was simply not a sufficient economic base to support a wide range of clients—it made a difference in terms of social acceptance. Potential clients had fewer worries in terms of stigma for their desire to change themselves; more important, doctors did not have to concern themselves with legal questions being raised about their practice.

Moreover, the medical literature for this period indicates that practitioners were continuing to hold on to the "reconstructive" label as representing the core of their practice, with aesthetic concerns coming later. Dr. Jae-Duk Yoo (1930–) of Yonsei University was interested in a wide range of medical subspecialties, and the overwhelming majority of his publications from this period tend to cluster around his concerns with skin grafts and tissue transplant.[58] Similarly, the first issue of the *Journal for the Korean Society of Plastic and Reconstructive Surgeons*, which appeared in late 1975, focuses on two broad categories of patients: those with congenital defects requiring repair and those with severe injuries sustained in daily life, with burn victims prominent among this second group.[59] This description, with perhaps a few exceptions, positions South Korean plastic surgery at this point as situated within the broad contours of Millard's postwar characterization of providing relief, if not necessarily within his more extreme views regarding the possibility of personal transformation.

Indeed, some of the most common surgeries at this time, as measured by the frequency of references in abstracts, had to do with ptosis, a congenital condition whereby "an inferior malposition of the upper eyelid margin relative to the pupil" occurs.[60] The condition may also be acquired with age, as folds of skin begin to accumulate on the upper eyebrow, interfering with and limiting one's range of vision. In more common parlance, the condition is sometimes characterized as analogous to "drooping eyelids," with the patient's vision left partially blocked or impaired, even with the eyes fully open. A child born with the condition would be an ideal candidate for surgical repair; in the decade of the 1960s, it is not difficult to find frequent references to it in Korean ophthalmology journals.

By the mid-1970s, South Korean plastic surgeons tended to view themselves very much as a community in transition, and one still possessing relatively modest goals. To offer a generalization, the aims of most procedures were still defined in terms of the repair of congenital deformities and defects or, cases of severe injury, placing the field as a whole within a reconstructive framework, one tied to the restoration of a patient to normal functioning. This was still, after all, a country without provision for any kind of comprehensive health coverage—this would be tentatively introduced beginning in 1977, and, following further reforms in 1989, would begin to reach a larger population—meaning that health care needed to identify and rely on the private consumer as the nation began to grow economically and reduce its dependence on international aid subsidies.

References to some form of the double eyelid surgery first began to appear in the Korean medical literature for this period, with the first abstracts emerging roughly in the mid-1970s. These cases are relatively few, however, and their medical interest is often confined not to the surgery itself but to the numerous complications associated with it. To summarize the tentative lineage we have constructed with respect to Japanese precedents, it should be clear that there is not a single procedure for "double eyelid" surgery but, rather, an entire cluster of related practices varying in degree with respect to the nature of the intervention and also with respect to the kinds of surgical tools employed. In the South Korean case, the desire to pursue epicanthoplasty, a complete removal of the epicanthic fold, has brought a great deal of attention to the issues of scarring and the proximity of the tear ducts.[61] Many of the earliest cases, appearing in dermatology and ophthalmology journals in the early 1970s, treat this kind of issue, generally concerned more with the aftermath of surgery, in other words, than its actual performance.

In his effort to establish as comprehensive a lineage as possible in *Asian Blepharoplasty* (1995), William Pai-Dei Chen goes so far as to offer separate lists for both the pre- and postwar periods, with the former, not surprisingly, dominated almost exclusively by the literature in Japanese.[62] The second list, of greater interest here, bears a strong resemblance to our earlier discussion concerning the postwar influx of military medicine, with several sites in the Anglo-American world—the Philippines, Singapore, and Hawaii—popping up early on and with even greater diversity appearing from about the early 1970s, by now including Taiwan, China, and Thailand.[63] South Korea, interestingly, does not make its first appearance until 1989, a relatively late date given our discussion.[64] This late inclusion is presumably driven by Chen's limitation in mainly pursuing titles published in English-language journals and, equally important, his desire to chronicle developments that mark a new point in practice.[65] In other words, the practice of some forms of eye surgery in South Korea almost certainly precedes Chen's recognition of 1989 as a start date, but the publications appear primarily in Korean-language journals, and the practice derived from a pool of existing surgical techniques, rather than breaking new ground.

To bring this discussion to its conclusion, the Korean article cited by Chen, with an international research team headed by Dr. Se-Min Baek, concerns the introduction of a nonincision surgical technique into the South Korean context.[66] A closer inspection of the report brings it roughly in line with our periodization, as the majority of the procedures in the sample took place between September 1981 and September 1985 at Inje hospital, with Dr. Baek representing part of a network that included his Japanese and American collaborators.[67] His pattern of citations proves revealing as well, as he recognizes the postwar developments taking place in Singapore and Japan as among those most relevant to his own work, the project of creating a supratarsal fold without the use of an incision. On this point, Dr. Baek is emphatic in his characterization of the role of the surgery within the region, stating that "the majority of patients who request a 'double fold' do not want to look more Western," preferring to conceive of the procedure as one bringing a more attractive look to the face within a local set of aesthetic norms.[68]

As Dr. Baek chooses to characterize the surgery in the language of the aesthetic, the consideration he grants to meeting patient wishes strongly emphasizes a move in this direction. At the same time, he places the procedure within a more complicated set of circumstances, acknowledging the different features common to his Korean patients, noting that there is not a single type of eyelid common to all.[69] If the emphasis here remains on an implied contrast between the Caucasian and Asian—or Oriental, to borrow the vocabulary of the title—this factor is certainly not one of the desired aims. For Baek, the aim is a pleasing result, one inherently satisfying to the patient and, more important, with a minimum of scarring or visible traces of the work done. The thrust lies in the direction of professionalization, the skillful performance of a difficult task rendered carefully and appropriately by a well-trained surgeon on behalf of a client.

With these claims, we see an understanding of the surgery that provides a contrast to Millard's version of radical ethnic transformation. In approximating the language of his patients, Dr. Baek invokes the newer vocabulary of the "round eye" as the desired aim, a form of visual appeal that can be equated with difference, while still lying well within the boundaries of Korean convention.

Moreover, Dr. Baek's challenge to the surgery characterizes it as an update to a known problem, a more visually appealing solution to a common issue. The focus here, in other words, is the reduction of scarring or swelling, not the fundamental alteration of identity, as the procedure is driven by the motivations and desires of a newer type of patient.

Where this discussion should go next is the legal and medical changes taking place in South Korea between the late 1970s and the early 1990s, with economic growth serving as one of the motivating forces enabling the development of a medical marketplace. Without significant legal change, the South Korean medical marketplace would not have become nearly as lucrative as it has, and we would not be able to identify it clearly with geographical precision. This argument ultimately aims to arrive in the Kangnam-gu district of Seoul, southeast of the Han River, where large clusters of private medical clinics are now clustered around the Apkujŏng and Sinsa subway stations.[70] This development represents a significant difference from the earlier period under discussion, with the eye surgery generally affiliated with hospitals, especially in terms of the availability of sophisticated equipment and highly trained personnel. Along with economic change, post-1987 democratic reforms meant that a new medical culture could emerge, one driven largely by private interests and the aggressive recruitment of patients as paying clients.

Health Insurance and the Provision of Health Care in South Korea (1977–1997)

This last remark should not suggest that the transformation of health care took place rapidly; indeed, many commentators have observed that the provision of wider forms of health coverage actually came late in terms of the South Korean developmental story. For the Park Chung Hee period, the 1977 health care law, often cited as marking the start of reform, was quite modest in its scope, requiring only that large firms with more than 500 employees begin to offer basic forms of coverage.[71] These figures affected only a limited percentage of the population, with follow-up refinements coming in 1979 and again in 1981, aiming to broaden the types of coverage available. For this period of nearly three decades, covering the first voluntary provision of health insurance to its extension to all firms with more than 100 employees (from 1963 to 1981), it is clear that the ROK government was acutely aware of its target demographic, consisting primarily of clusters of white-collar workers, bureaucrats, and a select number of industrial workers, those holding a significant investment in the state and its project. Health care remained highly selective in reaching its targets, a theme we have already witnessed in previous chapters in terms of evaluating access in terms of both class and regional differences.

If we focus here primarily on the 1977 effort at insurance reform, rather than its counterpart, the 1963 precedent, the issues remain similar, with the relationship between the state and corporate interests—here referring to the participation of *chaebŏl*—dictating the shape and extent of any proposed program. If this issue has emerged infrequently in preceding chapters covering this same span of time, especially Chapters 4 and 5, it serves now as a timely reminder, recognizing that both the family planning (from 1961 through 1985) and antiparasite campaigns (from 1969 through 1995) were conducted largely in the absence of state-driven mechanisms for collecting payment for the provision of these forms of health care.[72] This absence also helps to explain why many South Koreans continued to shop around, to invoke Dr. Jae-Mo Yang's metaphor, both on the grounds of familiarity and cost. In effect, the Park state enacted only stopgap measures to place health care on the books, offering little in the way of its enforcement or practical application, essentially deferring the issue.

Moreover, to return this discussion to the specific issue of surgery—regardless of whether reconstructive or aesthetic in its intent—there would be a conspicuous tension between those hoping to pursue a market-oriented approach and the general climate of South Korean health care, typically much more conservative.[73] This is another way of saying that although the late 1970s would witness varieties of eye surgery being performed with increasing skill and sophistication, the period did not necessarily welcome a new set of economic motives on the part of its practitioners. Even with the desire for greater profits, doctors still needed to create a niche for themselves, and they also needed accompanying legal and institutional changes to increase the cultural power of their practice. Many of the abstracts from this period continue to appear under the authority of large public hospitals and those affiliated with universities, indicating that major institutions were supporting this style of work without necessarily encouraging a culture of medical privatization, something that would not come along until the early 1990s.[74]

This use of the language of privatization anticipates the development of a new medical culture in perhaps too simple a fashion, using the abstraction of the market as a category to explain everything. In fact, the definition of the eyelid as an area subject to aesthetic concerns had not yet taken place, and this absence requires further investigation. Through the late 1970s and early 1980s, the reconstruction of the eyelid continued to center on either an illness such as cancer or, even more commonly, on congenital defects such as blepharoptosis, which we have discussed earlier, in which the eyelid droops prominently and requires correction. The shift to the aesthetic, while present in a limited number of cases, was not yet a major form of practice, with reconstructive work continuing to hold a dominant position. Again, this raises related issues of identity and concerns of self-perception, as well as the means of delivery, the form in which surgical services would be provided.

The "Underdevelopment" of Social Welfare: Creating Private Clinics

The private clinic, to use this category as a heuristic, held a very different set of associations as it changed over time, certainly as compared to its more positive connotations—specifically its association with affluence—in recent decades. As I have used this term previously, the implication connotes a specific type of referent, an area based outside a major city, suggesting a doctor working in isolation, without access to the same resources as his or her urban-based peers. This type of center, with a doctor working either alone or in combination with at most a partner or two, had to provide much of the primary care for rural Korea, even as many rural residents continued to meet basic medical needs at home, including the act of giving birth. The emphasis on these sites rested on providing the best care possible with a minimum of resources, meeting basic needs rather than providing any notion of specialist care. This distinction, as basic as it is, provides a valuable reminder of how rapid and thorough the recent transformation of South Korean health care has been. The emphasis on the word *private* here should suggest a lack or insufficiency, in contrast to any notion of exclusivity that might come into play.

So how and why would circumstances begin to change? The legal and institutional changes associated with health insurance reform (from 1977 through 1999) would hold major consequences for doctors, especially in terms of shaping their responses and motivations for making a career choice in a health-related field. In making the first tentative moves toward health care reform in the late 1970s, the Park Chung Hee government borrowed much of the governing logic for its decision from the case of Japan, even while continuing to be heavily influenced by American models of clinical practice.[75] According to Jong-Chan Lee, this resulted in an uncomfortable compromise, an approach that sought a middle ground between a completely private system based on fees generated by clients and a national health scheme directed by the state, with the latter of the two choices as one that might easily burden the government in times of economic crisis.[76] With the incremental expansion of the groups receiving coverage under the scheme, the tension between these conflicting impulses has grown, with private interests therefore starting to dominate by the late 1980s and early 1990s; in brief, a gap grew between fees deriving from the government scheme, with slow returns, and those from private patients, paying immediately on site.

The literature concerning South Korean social welfare policy has been remarkably reticent in failing to engage with the problem of health insurance, even while noting it as a dilemma, "a classic but puzzling question on the relationship between the capitalist development and the welfare state."[77] The general tendency has been to address the problem as one of the "underdevelopment of social welfare policy," with the authoritarian state dominating any discussion with labor and citizen's groups until as recently as the late 1980s. Or, to put this in other terms, South Korean civil society effectively made a bargain with the state to offer its cooperation and to defer social welfare, making concessions in exchange for economic growth that would benefit all. This model also helps to explain precisely why ROK health insurance is often characterized as late in its arrival, with the provision of national coverage not becoming a material reality until 1989. However, the danger here would be to read recent reforms as evidence of a fulfillment of the earlier delays, the completion of a promise made two to three decades previously.

Moreover, the emerging trend toward broader coverage should not be interpreted as a direct analogue to the capitalist terms of the American health market, or at least as it existed until recently, carrying notions of managed health care and the type of cost cutting expected of health maintenance organizations (HMOs). Rather, the South Korean health system has seen a vast expansion of the power of the individual doctor, with little or no regulation from a clinical standpoint, and this trend has continued to increase in the most recent decade (from 1997 through 2011). What this means in practical terms is that the incentive to practice private medicine has increased dramatically as the costs of working in the public sector have created pressures to limit costs within the South Korean public system. Not surprisingly, South Korean doctors able to bear the cost of setting themselves up in a clinical situation, whether individually or as part of a small collective, typically opt to do so, with the majority of these doctors taking on several specialties and with private medicine easily dominating the public sector. Simply put, the Korean doctor perceives this move as critical to economic survival, as specialties tend to offer the greatest opportunity for attracting funds and as private practice translates into less regulatory attention. Without this option, a doctor must rely on payment through national health insurance, which tends to be slow and does not cover many procedures.

This also means that the South Korean system is heavily oriented toward the delivery of specialist services, with the most lucrative transactions lying in the provision of pharmaceuticals and specialized forms of care. At least in this respect, South Korea's national health system is not that different from those of many other nations, where increasing sophistication has meant expensive diagnostic tests and sophisticated forms of instrumentation. In particular, the regulation of pharmaceuticals has meant a series of recent legal battles over the right to prepare and prescribe pharmaceuticals, as these are absolutely essential to the income of doctors. As for surgery, the turn toward private practice has meant a correspondingly higher degree of specialization, less clinical regulation, and ultimately a far more lucrative practice for those able to set up a private clinic.

Without sidetracking onto the numerous issues concerning the political strength of South Korean doctors, pharmacists, and medical workers as interest groups, it is worth mentioning here two major conflicts that have appeared within the last ten to fifteen years. First, Korean medical doctors and their TKM counterparts began to come into conflict in the mid-1990s with the growing power of TKM as a form of practice. Specifically, the government sought to extend the power to distribute pharmaceuticals—in this case, including the preparation of traditional remedies—to all pharmacists, a legal challenge that TKM practitioners sought to block.[78] Reserving the preparation and distribution of herbal remedies for their own exclusive use as a community, TKM practitioners have carved out a powerful space for themselves, especially with the professionalization that has allowed them to claim knowledge of both traditional practice as well as that of biomedicine.

Second, and even more relevant to our case here, a major strike of medical workers took place in 2000, with doctors, nurses, and medical support personnel creating a stalemate that would last much of the summer (from June through August) of that year. Here the issue centered precisely on questions of insurance reform, with many practitioners claiming that existing insurance schemes barely covered the costs of providing care. In this case, with a cycle of strikes continuing to the present, Korean medical workers have continued to resist national regulation, especially for most forms of clinical practice, instead shaping the process to reflect their interests. With no resolution in sight, the state has had to make many concessions to medical workers to maintain the functioning of the system, as imperfect as it is.

What this means for our story is that the shift toward the aesthetic, and away from reconstructive work, corresponds to the rapid growth of a newer style of private practice. There are exceptions to this observation, but it should not be surprising that while professional societies for maxillofacial and reconstructive surgery in Korea formed around the mid- to late 1970s, the majority of the comparable institutions for *aesthetic* plastic surgery would appear about a decade later, in the mid-1980s.[79] Again, this should not be read as simply the influx of money associated with economic growth overwhelming the medical marketplace but rather as the culmination of a lengthy series of negotiations between the developmental state and its partners, with the Park Chung Hee state and subsequent military governments approaching the problem incrementally. The question we will have to examine in subsequent sections concerns how this affects the practice of surgery, whether it remains intact or has become a very different type of procedure within this new setting.

In general, I will argue that the emphasis on the delivery of specialist services by South Korean doctors corresponds roughly to the growth of a new medical culture from the mid-1980s onward. That is, South Korean physicians have made a long-term pact with the state since the early 1960s, accepting less-than-ideal working conditions and less support from national health insurance in exchange for relative freedom and weaker forms of clinical regulation. In recent years, when the state has attempted to extend its oversight, both medical doctors and TKM practitioners have resisted fiercely, resorting to small-scale strikes and even direct appeals to the public. The growth of the private clinic, in contrast to the rural site as described here earlier, should now connote an elite, highly controlled space with a small group of specialists and a corresponding reliance on new technologies and sophisticated forms of practice. Since the early to mid-1990s, such specialists, especially those who claim expertise with respect to the body and aesthetic surgery, have tended to concentrate next to or around a highly specific geography in Seoul, especially the two subway stations of Sinsa and Apkujŏng, renowned as centers for plastic surgery.

Private Clinics and the Rise of Aesthetic Surgery (from the Early 1990s through the Present)

It is not sufficient to attribute the rapid growth of plastic surgery exclusively to the economic growth of the past three decades in South Korea (from 1980 through 2010); as I have argued here, the historical relationship between the state and the medical community has created an insurance scheme and regulatory climate in which doctors typically achieve the most lucrative practice in the form of surgical specialization, diagnostic tests, and the prescription of pharmaceuticals. Moreover, if we take Seoul as a case study, the physical geography of this type of practice is highly specific, clustered in certain locations just southeast of the Han River in the affluent area of Kangnam-gu. As recently as the second half of the 1970s, much of this land was still undeveloped, remote from downtown Seoul as an urban center; living close to the river often brought with it the potential for flooding and having one's home displaced. How and why have these sites developed in recent decades; more importantly for our story, how have these new clusters reconfigured the types of surgical practices that are being performed?

As open land available for sale and real estate speculation as recently as the early to mid-1970s, much of what now constitutes the Gangnam area underwent a rapid transition from farmland to urban space only within the last thirty to forty years. In particular, the population pressures in central Seoul (north of the river) made a move to the southern banks of the river highly desirable, and many of the new apartment complexes, like those situated in Chamsil (southeast Seoul), began to appear by about the mid-1970s. In the specific case of Chamsil, some apartments were allotted according to potential tenants' place in a queue, with family planning practices and the husband's willingness to undergo vasectomy figuring into the preference accorded to an individual family. Although remote from Seoul proper, in other words, Kangnam would be integrated with the growth of a more sophisticated transportation network via bus routes and the subway and quickly became a desirable address, both for residential living and for commercial settings. As the location of preference for a large number of plastic surgeons, there is no "natural" advantage to the site but instead a historically and culturally constructed association with new forms of affluence, the style of convenience and luxury associated with a narrative of self-transformation.

The origins of the Kangnam area surgical clinics followed with the settlement of the area as a prime location for real estate investors, although there was a significant time lag of ten to fifteen years between the first impulse of development and the arrival of the medical clinics as a significant commercial force in the surrounding area. According to an account by Hong Sung-Ho, a prominent practitioner, many of the first clinics selected traditional bases of commercial activity for their daily operations, including familiar sites such as Chongno (northern Seoul) and Myŏng-dong (north-central Seoul).[80] Both sites, north of the river, connote traditional sources of power and authority, and the latter, based close to the river, has long been associated with popular culture and the nearby film industry of Ch'ungmuro.[81] In Hong's account, the move to Kangnam took place only when the area established a reliable reputation for itself as a national trendsetter, a development that did not appear certain until at least the early 1990s. The present density, with Sinsa alone holding 163 plastic surgery clinics out of a national total of 728 (as of 2007), is primarily a product of the past two decades, with surgical specialization and a favorable climate for private practitioners.[82]

This level of density is by no means accidental, and if the geographical proximity to affluent areas represents a contributing factor, another—if highly speculative—has to do with what might be characterized as a "guild mentality," fostering a sense of community among practitioners. Marginalized from their many of their medical peers until recently, South Korean practitioners of plastic surgery have been enormously protective of their interests as a collective, using the media and the possibility of greater expression that came with recent cultural change to carve out and define a powerful niche for themselves as an economic entity. Moreover, if the desire to be situated in proximity suggests a communal ethic, it should not ignore the presence of competition, as this type of tension also exists. Especially with the export of South Korean popular culture, bringing with it the cosmetics industry and notions of personal transformation, practitioners have become aware of the potential to reach an international clientele. The Kangnam location is therefore not simply an issue of appealing to South Koreans but now also one of anticipating and accommodating the needs of foreign visitors.

We have to be careful of accepting this brief account as in any way "natural," coming as it does from a prominent representative of the industry, but Dr. Hong's remarks underscore the fact that practitioners were looking for a home base from as early as the 1980s, with advocates of private practice beginning to make a name for themselves. With the label "aesthetic" gaining acceptance, both popularly and professionally, from about the mid-1990s, it should not be surprising that these individuals would be looking for ways in which to consolidate their interests. From Dr. Hong's perspective, the intersection of collective interests made a good fit, as the area became known for its high-rise apartments and was typically associated with the growth of "new money" in a rapidly changing South Korea. If this account seems a bit too convenient, it does make sense that consumers with the disposable income and an inclination to pursue surgery would be looking for convenience and ease of access as well. And if this account cannot explain the clusters around the two subway stations in particular, it at least offers the beginning of an outline in which the concentration of new wealth was followed by service industries catering to specifically this type of clientele.

Moreover, the type of physician likely to settle in this area was aware of the possibilities of self-promotion, as the age of the "celebrity surgeon" coincided roughly with the arrival of the plastic surgery industry as a major commercial force. That is, even as public awareness was growing, a small number of surgeons made use of the media to publicize their concerns, advocating on behalf of the interests of their community. Starting in the 1980s, both television and print media began to refer more frequently to a select handful of these individuals, willing to present themselves as the public face of an industry that was rapidly gaining a foothold, with professional respectability to follow.[83] If the large clinics in Sinsa should be associated primarily with the 1990s, we can think of the decade immediately preceding in terms of a wider distribution of such clinics in a cluster of urban areas—as already noted, based primarily in Chongno and Myŏng-dong—with a corresponding trend in the growth of media coverage and with plastic surgeons taking a proactive stance toward attempts to regulate their work.

If plastic surgery was at this time framed largely in terms of its appeal to a domestic market, its aims intensified with the added pressure of growing economic competition at the domestic level and with the Asian financial crisis of 1996 through 1997.[84] The crisis, associated largely in South Korea with the intervention of the IMF (International Monetary Fund), with the organization becoming the subject of a great deal of dark humor in the South Korean context, brought change to how surgery could be packaged.[85] That is, if plastic surgery as a whole continued to be viewed as a luxury by many, something associated with a growing affluence, it also became a necessity to some, a set of practices that might provide one with a decided advantage in the job market. With this approach, surgery in the second half of the 1990s became a tool for self-realization, no longer perceived simply in terms of a person's self-concept but now critical to the lengthy process of acquiring and keeping a job.

To further illustrate the geographical specificity of these trends, we can appeal to the statistics for this most recent period, covering the years from 2000 through 2005, focusing on the location and relative density of clinics based in the city of Seoul. For the year 2000, there were just under 5,000 clinics, with these figures climbing to reach a rough figure of 6,500 by the year 2005, reflecting an increase of about 30 percent.[86] Of these clinics, 935 were located in Kangnam-gu, providing a total of just over 600 hospital beds.[87] These figures tend to reinforce two observations: Kangnam has by far the greatest density of private health care clinics for the city of Seoul, and it generally provides few on-site facilities, meaning that the majority of the work is performed on an outpatient basis. These figures do not refer to plastic surgery exclusively but rather the entirety of the range of clinics; still, this portrait offers support for the growing economic and cultural power of commercial health care, especially in its private form.

This trend of increase, along with other new uses of eye surgery, helps to explain the embrace of the aesthetic hinted at earlier in this chapter. The reconstructive context still had its appeal in cases of obvious necessity, but the overwhelming majority of cases shifted to the possibility of realizing the client's desired self-image through surgery, whether for personal or professional reasons. The venue would most likely be one of the new types of urban clinics as outlined here, with the work done on an outpatient basis and performed using the latest available technologies, especially the laser. The diversity of possible surgeries—again, there are a wide variety of approaches reflected under the broad category of blepharoplasty—would be packaged primarily in terms of the possible enhancements to the client's personal and professional development, simplifying the choice by focusing on a cluster of desired results. In this sense, the claims made by Millard in the early 1950s, while not replicated, appear in the form of similar tropes: The key difference here is that the surgery can make a much stronger case for taking place in a genuinely "Korean" context—with both Korean practitioners and patients.

Having said this, transnational exchange between South Korea and the United States was quite extensive by the early 1990s, whether measured in terms of short-term educational exchange, long-term immigration, or, more important, the exchange of aesthetic norms and images taken from popular culture. This has an impact on our story here in particular in the relationship between a significant Korean American community and their relatives in South Korea, with the ease of travel and new forms of social media serving to increase the frequency and the impact of contact. For example, some medical anthropologists have looked at the eye surgery in terms of its impact on the formation of a specifically Asian American identity, arguing that the American market would become a key factor as young people traveled back and forth between these different contexts.[88] This point is particularly relevant with respect to young Koreans and their Korean American counterparts, as short-time exchange—especially in the summer, for education and cultural contact—has become extremely popular, corresponding to the growth of South Korean affluence.

As we return to the issue of the surgery and its revised meanings within the last two decades, this issue of cultural exchange remains on the table, although we will focus primarily on the reconfiguration of the South Korean medical marketplace, as outlined in the previous sections. We are therefore concerned with the eye surgery as it plays out within these new clinical settings: private hospitals set up primarily for the purpose of performing aesthetic procedures, often for a combination of personal and professional aims. Even with insurance reform, many of these surgeries would not be eligible for medical coverage, but the issue of payment was far less of a concern in a South Korea that achieved a $10,000 per capita gross national product (GNP) as of 1996, an accomplishment receiving a great deal of media coverage. In fact, part of the appeal of the surgery might be interpreted in precisely this light, with the ability to pay for a transformative experience outside of the traditional medical system attesting even more to its special character.

Asian Blepharoplasty (post-1997): Mobilizing Aesthetic Practice and Style

The claim of providing a personal transformation, even if not necessarily a complete bridging of racial or ethnic lines, explains in part why Millard's work has remained central to the issue, even if enormously controversial. In particular, his surgical work on the supratarsal fold continues to generate a large number of citations in English-language publications, depending on whether a surgeon follows Millard's practice or adopts an alternative method. Remember that Millard's procedure originally concerned the upper eyelid and specifically the decision to use sutures to create a fold or to create the same effect through the removal of excess tissue.[89] The range of possible practices has greatly expanded in intervening years, to the point where there are now many procedures using incisions as well as those without, a key factor in controlling and limiting the visibility of any subsequent scarring. Another issue is whether to perform related procedures, such as the epicanthoplasty, the complete removal of the epicanthic fold.

In other words, preferences and styles for eye surgery have undergone dramatic changes, and "Asian blepharoplasty" contains within it a plurality, a number of related practices under its broad rubric. If the motivations and enabling factors for this development include the economic progress made by South Korea during the mid-1980s, along with the legal and cultural changes enabling the growth of private clinics, it is also useful to look at material practice, with the clinics adopting new technologies and a range of options to meet the needs of clients. These are frequently South Korean young people, who may have traveled and have been exposed to a wide variety of images before coming to the decision to undergo surgery. If we are going to characterize this revised style of practice "aesthetic," we need to look briefly at how this translates into the actual procedures performed in clinical settings.

Millard's original language (1955) invoked the conception of a "round eye" in pushing for the surgery, with the creation or simulation of a double fold in the upper eyelid approximating a "Western" visage. Even from this early standpoint, Millard and other practitioners understood that there was great diversity among their Asian patients, with some members of the population possessing a natural fold and with a wide range of variation in the crease of the upper eyelid. Since the period of intense interest generated approximately fifty to fifty-five years ago (from 1955 through 1960), surgical techniques and forms of instrumentation have changed dramatically, and the introduction of laser surgery and control of local anesthesia has made blepharoplasty in particular a far more sophisticated form of work. For our story here, what matters now is how the surgery has been reconceived in the South Korean context within the last two decades, especially within the setting of the private clinic.

Redefining the "Round Eye"?

Even as there remains a fair amount of diversity in terms of surgical practice, it is possible to make generalizations about the transformation of stylistic preferences in the Korean context, with certain tropes starting to appear more regularly. In particular, dissatisfaction with common blepharoplasty, along with related anatomical claims about the surface of the upper eyelid—whether real or perceived—have led to the popularity of a number of follow-up or accompanying procedures in many cases. Frequently, this translates into blepharoplasty (reshaping of the area around the eye) being linked with epicanthoplasty, an attempt either to remove completely, or to at least minimize, the presence of the epicanthic fold in the upper eyelid area. In turn, the epicanthic fold is often associated with a less prominent upper eyelid crease, although the link is not a necessary one, as the two features remain distinct. In any event, it is a simple matter to find surgical abstracts from the last two decades detailing updates to the surgery in South Korea, often building on methods previously developed in Japan.

By itself, epicanthoplasty is considered something of a risk, and many surgeons will not attempt it because of the proximity of the tear ducts and the possibility of damaging the drainage these provide to the eyes. This factor has not diminished its popularity in Asia, but surgeons do have to caution patients about the possible risks, and one popular plastic surgery clinic in Seoul estimates that it performs the epicanthoplasty in only about one-quarter of its encounters with the eye and the surrounding area.[90] Along with the difficulty of the procedure, scarring of the upper eyelid surface also represents a genuine concern, and here we see the intersection of the pragmatic and the aesthetic, with South Korean surgeons mobilizing their expertise to claim mastery of this difficult area. There are a number of possible ways to obscure or hide scars, if any should appear, and Korean surgeons have become very adept at this art.

In addressing this concern, Korean surgeons have turned to the legacy of practice available to them, with Junichi Uchida's (1962) publication representing a particularly influential model, precisely because of its claim to minimize external scarring. In effect, the use of epicanthoplasty in the South Korean context, though viewed as something of a radical procedure in many other settings, has necessitated greater attention to this issue. Publishing in the *British Journal of Plastic Surgery*, Uchida described using a series of silk and catgut sutures to connect the levator muscle and fix it to the tarsal plate, achieving the desired visual effect.[91] Although the procedure is not duplicated in precisely the same fashion in its contemporary usage, it is frequently cited as a precedent, with modifications made to fit the preferences of Korean surgeons working since about the early 1990s. Thus, references to a "modified Uchida procedure" appear quite frequently in surgical abstracts, with this pattern reinforcing the pattern of an ongoing exchange of ideas and practice between the Korean and Japanese medical communities.

The Uchida precedent has been influential because of its close attention to aesthetic concerns, particularly the issue of visible scarring. If Millard attempted to disguise the effects of his work with a "Z plasty," burying a scar within nearby folds of skin—with Z indicating the rough outline of the fold—Uchida was even more successful in adopting a similar type of strategy, often described as a "split V-W plasty," or sometimes taking the form of a "V-Y plasty." Again, the alphabetic references here refer to the approximate shape of the area of skin put to use, with the natural creases in the area used to obscure any traces of surgery. Even as Korean surgeons have modified Uchida's work, taking a variety of stances on the question of what kind of incision need be made, as well as the extent of and size of the skin fold, the presumed similarities between Korean and Japanese anatomical features continue to make his work a popular model for this kind of procedure.

This emphasis on the reduction, if not the complete elimination, of any signs of scarring underscores the heightening of aesthetic concerns within the last two to three decades in South Korea (from 1980 to 2010). Rather than allowing this concern to become a problem, however, Korean practitioners have mobilized their expertise in these problematic areas, making the epicanthoplasty, treated as something of a risk in many other nations, far more common. In terms of stylistic preferences as well, the vocabulary used to describe the shape and placement of the eye socket has shifted, with the generic term "round eyes" receiving further qualification. Specifically, many surgeons in recent years have criticized the surgical work of their predecessors not for its technique but for its effects, drawing the skin tightly around the eyes, creating a "sharp" look, with extremely taut skin. Similar accounts of such an effect describe a "surprised" look to the eye, again due to the effects of stretching the skin. In contrast, practitioners are now careful to consult with patients in making presurgical choices, with a preference for "big eyes."

What this language means precisely can be difficult to qualify, but essentially it means a "softer" look to the skin immediately surrounding the eyes, an effect achieved—or so many practitioners now like to claim—by combining blepharoplasty with epicanthoplasty, with the added procedure helping to achieve the desired result. In the South Korean context at least, there is now a strong relationship between these two acts, even if the relationship remains one primarily of association rather than necessity. Moreover, on this point of "big eyes," the language refers to both the width of the eye and the height of the eye in its presentation, this language having largely replaced the previous vocabulary aiming for "round eyes." To cite a common example from the present, the BK Dongyang plastic surgery clinic in Seoul offers consumers its "Producing Big Eyes" program, with a variety of procedures and options from which to choose.[92] Whether "big eyes" connote "Westernization" per se remains an open issue, but, from a surgical standpoint, the degree and types of intervention have increased, as have the diversity of options available to a client.

This last point deserves further comment, especially in terms of a prominent clinic like the BK Donyang, among the most famous in South Korea. Rather than focusing on the problems and difficulties with eye surgery, practitioners have quite astutely mobilized the anatomical differences between the "Asian" and "Western" eyelid to construct an entire menu of possible options, with individual items catering to specific features. Again, the use of blepharoplasty (reshaping) along with epicanthoplasty has become fairly common in South Korea; and BK specifically mobilizes this combination as one designed for handling both the vertical and horizontal dimensions of the eye socket. Other possibilities include specialized treatments for ptosis (drooping folds of skin in the area), thereby alleviating the effect of "sleepy" or "tired" eyes, and of course they take into consideration the degree of intervention with respect to any incisions rendered. The "big eye," if it is to be distinguished from its predecessor, the "round eye," differs less in appearance than in the degree of control afforded, with individual features and selection criteria determined by the client in consultation with a specialist.

This policy holds for the full range of the lifespan as well, as clinics such as BK Dongyang no longer cater to a limited clientele and aim very ambitiously to meet the needs of both younger patients and their seniors. For the latter group, there is an increasingly specialized subset of options designed to treat the combined effects of environment and aging. These include procedures for treating any darkening of the skin and wrinkles in the area of the eye socket, as well as blepharoplasty for either the upper or lower portion of the eyelid, targeting specific areas for a tightening of the skin. Not specific to any age group but presumably aimed at attracting repeat business, there are also procedures for those dissatisfied with a previous surgery. Forming part of the BK's "revisional and reconstructive" program, this type of work underscores the desire of medical professionals to build a long-term relationship, whereby clients will need to return at regular intervals for surgical maintenance. The older model of a treatment that resolves a problem carries with it a certainty that practitioners still hope to convey, but they also recognize the need for building a practice that involves multiple visits, at least potentially.

And to offer a generalization, the stylistic preference for a particular type of eye now tends to accommodate a wider range of possibilities within this loose conception of "big eyes." In the recent volume, *Cosmetic Surgery of the Asian Face* (2005), the editors, McCurdy and Lam, urge that "patients should not be condemned to construction of the classic 'westernized' eyelid," a reference to the style of the early postwar period.[93] Similarly, other authors characterize this look as appearing alternatively "aggressive" or "sharp," but there is a general consensus around the notion that surgical technique has improved dramatically and that a patient's individual preferences should be respected. If the South Korean context frequently encourages blepharoplasty in conjunction with epicanthoplasty as a possible combination, there remains a willingness to consult with patients about their individual aims and desires. The notion of a menu includes everything from procedures as minimal as the introduction of a palpebral fold to more involved forms of intervention.

The growth of this culture has not come without its social costs, of course, and this topic has become the subject of increasing attention from scholars and activists. The documentary anthology *If You Were Me*, 2, a series of documentary shorts commissioned around the broad theme of human rights in South Korea, includes several segments pertaining to the conjoined themes of body image and plastic surgery.[94] One of these clips covers the procedure to sever the frenum, the tissue connecting the tongue to the floor of the mouth, surgery that Korean parents occasionally ask for their children in the belief that it will improve their English pronunciation through greater mobility. Another covers the difficulty faced by a young woman who is concerned about her appearance, affecting not only her school performance and relations with peers but also her potential on the job market after completing school. As for a broader sociological take on this issue, Elizabeth Lee's *Good for Her* (2004) contains a number of interviews with South Korean women between their twenties and forties, attempting to capture their responses to the development and availability of this culture.[95]

Lee's take on the emergence of the culture opts primarily for a feminist perspective, aiming to situate the surgical marketplace within the patriarchal system of South Korean employers and an increasingly competitive job market. Although her discussion of changing conceptions of beauty is interesting in itself, what the documentary really contributes is a rich sense of how plastic surgery in general ties into the availability of what appears to be a form of empowerment, ironically enabled by Korean women gaining access to better incomes and forms of employment in the last two to three decades. For our interest here, the eyes and the immediate visibility of the face, the film is accurate in its portrayal of the overlap between appearance and employment in contemporary South Korea, as well as the increasing prominence of a film and popular culture industry that has expanded beyond Korea to become both a regional and global presence. That is to say, if Western images and conceptions of beauty have tended to dominate in the past, South Korea has absorbed these, only to emerge with its own hybrid pop culture that now influences young people in locations ranging from Beijing to the urban centers of Southeast Asia.

If space permitted here, we could easily extend this discussion to include more recent trends in medical tourism (post-1997) as promoted by the South Korean government, and their corresponding effects on neighbors in the surrounding region. Even without this material, though, the basic point should be clear: Whatever their motives for choosing eye surgery, South Korean patients are drawing on a practice with deep historical ties, particularly to the region surrounding the peninsula and more specifically referring to the domestic context, associated with the practice of reconstructive surgery stemming from the Korean War. Dr. Millard was hardly alone in learning from his experience with Korean patients and American GIs, and it is possible to place other specialties in this context as well, including hand surgery and vascular surgery. The subsequent rise of a medical marketplace in South Korea, while tied to changes in mores and practices, has equally to do with the logic of the health insurance industry and its regulations governing practitioners, encouraging specialization at the social cost of unnecessary surgeries.

Conclusion: Challenging Developmental Expectations

Learning to Identify: Negotiating a "South Korean" Medical Practice?

In October 2005, I conducted an interview with the assistance of Dr. Kim Ok-Ju of Seoul National University, with the subject, Dr. Choo Kun Won, detailing his past as a medical student under Japanese colonialism in the late 1930s and early 1940s (he was a 1943 graduate of Keijo Imperial University).[1] Dr. Choo was one of a handful of Korean elites at Keijo Imperial University, and I was particularly interested in his evaluation of its medical pedagogy, as well as his recollection of treatment at the hands of Japanese colleagues. Two things in particular struck me during the interview, the first having to do with Dr. Choo's personal identity. Much to my surprise, he had largely positive things to say about his education and exhibited few signs of resentment toward the colonial regime. His pride at completing the medical program at Keijo was conspicuous, even while never challenging his basic sense of being a Korean. Succeeding on the terms of a Japanese imperial system during a difficult time may or may not have created personal and professional difficulties for him in the aftermath of World War II, but this was clearly a concern that did not have a strong impact on him.

The second point had to do with his use of the American military presence as a rhetorical dividing line, a marker of change. In Dr. Choo's estimation, the culture of medicine began to change almost immediately after August 1945, marking a sharp break with what came before. Given the duration of the interview, his age, and the vagaries of memory, Dr. Choo's recollections here were no doubt shaped by a desire to remember events in a particular way, with the arrival of the Americans marking a transition that resonates today. Still, his conviction is less interesting for its rhetorical force than for the underlying tensions that it stirs up with respect to Japanese colonialism and its accompanying models of biomedicine and public health. Even as Dr. Choo has successfully negotiated the complex life of a former colonial subject who continues to identify as a Korean, before becoming an elite doctor in South Korea, he recognizes at some level the need to break his career into distinct intervals.

Much of the medical historiography for South Korea continues to follow this trend, with the intervening period of Japanese rule representing a significant problem for any attempt to frame a national history. Advocates of the Yonsei University and Severance Hospital approach tend to favor tropes of duration, with the twin institutions tracing a common set of origins back to the late nineteenth century and the accompanying Horace Allen story of missionary origins.[2] This approach sets as its priorities persistence and struggle in the face of external rule, adding luster to the story, an aim reflected in the slogan frequently mobilized on behalf of the university, "the First and the Best."[3] In contrast, Seoul National University celebrates its origins in the aftermath of *haebang* ("liberation," referring to August 15, 1945), thereby claiming for itself the status of an institution created specifically by and for Koreans.[4] This narrative handles the Japanese question of influence rather deftly and tends to marginalize the role of the American military presence by emphasizing a rapid transition to Korean rule, with the Korean War to follow shortly thereafter.

In both cases, historiographical issues are handled through a careful manipulation of the chronology, deferring on far more complex issues of identity and professional practice. While I cannot claim to have answered these questions definitively, I have emphasized that medical practice, for elites like Dr. Choo—along with many others who have appeared in these pages, such as the ambitious cardiac surgeons Drs. Lee Chang-Bum and Lee Young-Gyun, as well as prominent public health experts, such as Drs. Kwon E Hyock and Yang Jae-Mo—allowed for the simultaneous practice and embodiment of overlapping forms of identity as South Korea constructed its emerging national story. This observation holds true for personal identity, as well as professional practice, meaning that South Korean physicians, doctors, and nurses continued to rely on the practice of "Japanese" medicine for some time, at least certainly from the perspective of external observers, if not necessarily these actors themselves. Moreover, this is not a story of benevolent health care divorced from local politics but that of a new nation deeply enmeshed in an emerging economy of international aid, forced to make difficult choices and compromises that resonate today. In both their practice and the forms of intervention they undertake, South Korean medical practitioners are clearly a product of the historical circumstances in which they found themselves.

As for corresponding question of self-perception and representation, this is a much more difficult set of issues, and I seldom had the opportunity to frame, let alone direct, this style of inquiry to senior Korean doctors, physicians, and nurses in the course of my research. Still, it is worth considering the work of Tessa Morris-Suzuki, who suggests that the repatriation scheme in 1945 did not fit the needs of many ethnic Koreans, particularly those born and raised in Japan, who did not necessarily identify with a "return" to Korea as enforced by the GHQ occupation. Morris-Suzuki further complicates these issues of identification by noting that international recognition of South Korea (*Taehan Min'guk*) in 1948 did not necessarily accelerate the process.[5] The creation of an independent nation implied a permanent division that many could not accept and was packaged along with the close sponsorship of its American patron, which some also found troubling.

According to her figures, identification with the new nation only began to take place in increments, becoming more common by the late 1950s, and this process approximates what one might expect with such a difficult and uncomfortable transition. In contrast to the neat division proposed by Dr. Choo, the creation of an independent South Korea required considerable time and effort. What these chapters have attempted to do is to illustrate this process of cultural transformation in rich material detail, especially through the mobilization of the "new": more specifically, new forms of medical pedagogy, new institutions reconstituted from the fragments of previous Korean institutions (along with a significant legacy of Japanese influence), and new public health campaigns designed to elicit the participation of desired target demographics. If there was tension among these competing models and practices, there was equally a fair degree of success in the end, as South Korea began to provide a baseline form of health care to a greater portion of its population roughly two to three decades after achieving its independence (from 1948 to 1977). At the same time, it did so by allowing practitioners to carry out many of the same exploratory impulses and medical practices previously explored by Japanese colonial officials.

Managing Developmental Expectations

If this process of eclectic borrowing and nation building had much to do with reestablishing a stable sense of identity, moreover, it also had to do with managing domestic and international expectations regarding what might be accomplished with the considerable financial and technical resources the ROK would receive as a Cold War partner.[6] Indeed, South Korean aid organizations frequently mobilize the trope of the nation having successfully completed its transformation, going from an aid recipient in the 1950s to an aid giver in the 1990s, implying the fulfillment of a developmental path.[7] Missing from this narrative, however, is the difficult and painful work associated with this transition, if in fact it has been "completed" in any sense; it more likely represents an ongoing process. It is understandable why South Korean governmental bodies and NGOs might favor this brand of narrative, as images from this period—especially early impressions formed in the aftermath of the Korean War—continue to shape coverage of the nation, creating lasting perceptions that are difficult to overcome.

*The Minnesota Project (1954–1962) and the National Medical Center (*Kungnip Ŭiryowŏn*) (1958–1968)*

For medicine specifically, this path can be described first in terms of the nation's ability to educate its own nurses and doctors and, more important, to employ them productively following completion of their degrees. With its heavy emphasis on Confucian values and higher education, South Korea did not experience much difficulty in recruiting students to medicine, and the production of larger numbers of Western-trained professionals began almost immediately, even preceding independence in August 1948. Keeping these professionals in South Korea was a very different story, and for a long time, South Korea—much like the Philippines and other developing countries—would be a net exporter of its best graduates, sending them abroad through international labor migration. Famously, Park Chung Hee sent a group of miners (for the coal industry) and nurses to West Germany in the early 1960s in a show of solidarity with a close "Free World" ally. Moreover, changes to American immigration law in 1965 widened access to immigration from Asia, meaning that South Korean doctors and nurses could now choose to stay in the United States on a long-term basis following graduation. This had not been a significant problem with the Minnesota Project (from 1954 through

1962), with the vast majority of its trainees returning from their study abroad in Minneapolis.

The transitional period marking the handover from the Rhee Syngman government to that of Park Chung Hee (from April 1960 to March 1961) witnessed some of the greatest turmoil in recent South Korean history, and these events provided an opportunity for not only Korean but also international participation. In an account of the National Medical Center's history assembled by members of the Scandinavian consortium, we learn that the hospital became directly involved with events in the street, receiving "within a few hours, 250 severe casualties for treatment," an unexpected crisis that staff members handled capably.[8] In meeting "this test in a way which was highly admired by Koreans and foreigners alike," the NMC cemented its reputation with the population and, more important, the government, giving the project the chance to continue beyond its awkward period of transition, something that Minnesota would fail to do.[9] Still, the economy was not yet sufficiently developed to provide full employment for graduates of the ambitious project, leaving an export model as the primary option.

In the case of Minnesota, doctors and nurses in training—regardless of whether based in Seoul or Minneapolis—already had a position waiting for their return, whereas with the NMC the transition from Scandinavian staff to Korean control took place at a much reduced pace. This factor, along with economic realities, provided fewer opportunities and incentives for highly trained medical graduates to remain at home. As a result, there was an outflow of medical personnel for much of the 1960s, with both doctors and nurses moving abroad. In the case of nurses, these hard-working, well-trained Koreans earned for themselves an enviable reputation, so much so that certain countries began recruitment campaigns, specifically targeting groups of South Korean nurses. The nations in question would include the United States, West Germany, and Canada, with the Scandinavian countries also joining in, attempting to direct this traffic to their own advantage.[10] In fact, the NMC hospital board even had to intervene, requesting that home country sponsors cease their programs of recruitment, as this activity hindered efforts at promoting the growth of a domestic medical community.[11]

This indicates that the collective effects of the two major pedagogy programs, the Minnesota Project and the NMC, were heavily mediated by material circumstances, with the domestic economy and labor migration figuring prominently among the factors. Certainly the degree of professionalization in

South Korean medicine witnessed a transition beginning from about the late 1950s, but this tended to overlap with a corresponding out-migration of many of these graduates, with both doctors and nurses frequently citing the United States among their destinations of choice. Although the image of the Korean doctor living abroad never reached that of the Filipino expatriate nurse or doctor—another community with a consistent pattern of labor migration to the United States—there are large clusters of such individuals situated close to major American biomedical research sites even today, with Bethesda, Maryland, constituting one such example of an elite Korean expatriate community, given its proximity to Washington, DC, and more importantly, the NIH (National Institutes of Health).[12]

To sustain a domestic medical community, two things had to happen, along with the economic development that fueled much of the transition. First, South Korean health professionals had to reach out to a much larger proportion of the population, and they managed this in part through the massive public health campaigns of the Rhee and Park periods. If tuberculosis and leprosy were major concerns at the end of the 1950s, the enthusiastic mobilization of the *Taehan Kajok Kyehoek Hyŏphoe* (family planning) and the *Kisaengch'ung Pangmyŏl Hyŏphoe* (antiparasite) organizations made it difficult to ignore the state's investment in the individual's health (*kŏn'gang*) by late in the following decade, now recast as a matter of overlapping personal and national interest. Second, the system of payment for health care had to change dramatically, and this transformation took place over three decades (from 1963 to 1989), with hospitals gradually enforcing new standards for payment and with health insurance coverage ensuring at least a minimum of care.

The Traffic in Bodies: Redefining "Health" for a Domestic Audience

This collective activity was not simply about building a medical community but also about reassuring the South Korean people that the ROK government was willing and capable of fulfilling its end of the social contract in the form of social welfare, combining nation building with a strong dose of paternalism. The images that circulated in the United States in the aftermath of the Korean War told Americans a comforting Cold War story about their nation's concern for a "Free World" neighbor in need, one requiring assistance and sufficient time in which to rebuild. Although there is room to speculate about the extent to which Koreans knew of this story and, in turn, its effects on them, South Korean popular imagery from the late 1950s onward tells a different, if related, tale, one about assuming one's duties with respect to maintaining personal health and the nation. Especially with the arrival of a new decade, the message of public health in South Korea became an aggressive one, with clear target figures to be achieved through self-discipline.

Health and the Nation

Both the family planning and antiparasite campaigns extended the penetration of biomedicine beyond its previous boundaries, confined to the controlled spaces of hospital sites and clinics. This is not to say that South Koreans did not continue to consult with traditional practitioners and to purchase ingredients for traditional remedies in the outdoor market. These forms of practice remained enormously popular and, in fact, essential, particularly because much of the country remained a rural, agrarian society that embraced medical pluralism. But now these same individuals encountered biomedicine much more frequently in their dealings with the state, whether in the form of reporting for military service or attending school or even within the family unit, in the course of reproduction. Here the message was about the potential afforded through a rhetoric of self-control and regulation; moreover, there were considerable incentives attached to compliance.

At the beginning of FP (1964), the goals mobilized were still abstract, motivated by a notion that collective action would be beneficial at the national scale, but increasingly these aims took a concrete, material form. A famous stamp issued to commemorate family planning month reflects this trend, with a family from the past fading away, outlined in gray, with their more modern counterparts shaded in the foreground in tones of a darker aqua blue. The former group contains six members—four children, along with two parents—while the latter takes the form of a nuclear family: two parents and their two children. What is more important here, comparatively, are the two family residences, with the thatched roof of a village hut giving way to a modern house, a warm, stable structure consisting of the desired combination of newer materials: brick, wood, and concrete. If the reality was that most South Koreans later lived in high-rise apartments, not stand-alone homes, this was no problem, as compliance with family planning also placed individuals at a greater advantage in the lottery for such new residences, beginning in the mid-1970s.

Through the circulation of new publications such as *kajŏng ui pŏt* ("Happy Home," 1968) and *Kŏn'gang* ("Health," 1973), magazines associated with the FP and antiparasite campaigns respectively, South Koreans could easily learn about the increasingly diverse lifestyle choices available to them, with material goods figuring prominently, shifting with a general trend toward urbanization and the move to apartments. Moreover, both magazines contained numerous ads for pharmaceuticals and related products, taking the purchase of these goods out of the traditional marketplace and repackaging them in commercially available form. Again, this is not to deny the critical role of the traditional practitioner within Korean culture, but, especially during the first two decades following the Korean War, the activity of manufacturing and selling medical-related products came to be associated increasingly with the pharmacy and the biomedical doctor.

Kŏn'gang, in particular, would focus less on material goals than *kajŏng ui pŏt*, but neither was the publication simply a bland compilation of statistics and public health information, the type of information that might easily be found in an annual report. Rather, the magazine sought to engage Koreans at the level of useful tips for better living, leading the reader to recognize how and why these facts might be of interest. At times, this could make for rather intense reading, as was the case with the feature article, "Why Are Parasites Frightening?" (*"Kisaengch'ung ŭn wae musŏun'ga?"*), appearing prominently in one of the first issues.[13] At the same time, other articles covered topics such as how to adapt one's lifestyle to changes in the weather or seasons, as well as how to deal with more common household pests, such as mosquitoes. In other words, the motivation underlying the publication, beyond its surface of providing a public health message, was one of convenience and control, establishing the basis for a more comfortable and safer environment that could be achieved throughout the reader's home and neighborhood.

In both of these health campaigns, this kind of appeal to pragmatic self-interest helped to mediate between the state and individual, making it difficult to view the Park period as exclusively one of top-down control. Rather, it was a positive message of bettering the nation, leaving behind the vocabulary of "reconstruction" and embracing an optimistic future. South Koreans, especially women in the case of the FP campaign, joined in eagerly to help create an incipient brand of nationalism in which to participate was to be faithful to the state's message, while also furthering one's own chances. And it was not hard to see results, as more apartment houses were being constructed rapidly by late in the decade of the 1960s, with the hastily constructed wooden homes along the Han River starting to disappear. If the tenuous connections between these developments were not always obvious, there were always more posters, pamphlets, and slogans to reinforce the point: Consent to these campaigns would lead to a better life.

To cite the work of Ruth Rogaski, the spread of antipest campaigns in a public setting, along with the display of a banner concerning a health concern, was actually not new in much of East Asia. Instead, what was new was the mobilization of a modern vision of a progressive biomedicine, one that could resolve the problems in question. Although Koreans were familiar with the problem of rats and other pests, with eradication campaigns echoing similar Chinese campaigns, the use of DDT and more powerful pesticides in the streets constituted a new development. Moreover, for much of the Park period and well into the early 1980s, the question of funding this new style of medical treatment and related public health was deferred, with the prospect of health insurance treated only nominally (in 1963 and 1977). For its part, the state provided as it could, with international partners helping to assume much of the burden, effectively subsidizing much of the public health activity.[14]

"Mixed Medicines": Post-1987 and the ROK Health System

With a strong emphasis on biomedicine and the benefits it can provide, one of the more surprising developments post-1987 has been the emergence of a radically reconfigured form of traditional practice, a TKM with a claim to a rich historical legacy, yet with access to the tool kit of the scientific method. If the story has been almost exclusively about biomedicine to this point, it should not neglect the legacy of traditional practice, which in multiple ways continues to inform the practice and habits of South Koreans. The scholar Sokhieng Au has recently mobilized the term *mixed medicines* to capture the plural medical character of Cambodia, a society where many accept and make use of a diversity of medical practices.[15] The term can cover a wide range of East and Southeast Asian social contexts, fitting comfortably with Vietnam and China, among others. If the analogy to the South Korean case feels a bit unusual, it is perhaps because of the implicit developmental judgment, with many arguing that the ROK has somehow completed its developmental experience, one distinct from that of its regional neighbors.

It is precisely against this brand of exceptionalism that I direct these remarks, and in this sense, the analogy between South Korea and its Southeast and Northeast Asian regional neighbors proves quite fitting. Yes, traditional practice in today's South Korea represents a radically reconfigured and much more powerful form of practice because it has successfully carried out its own professionalization scheme (from 1965 through the early 1980s), such that those wishing to receive degrees must first earn the equivalent of a Western medical degree, in addition to studying the underlying principles of *Hanŭihak*. Kyunghee University houses perhaps the most famous of these programs, but there now are a number of other well-respected programs, with the TKM degree itself representing a well-established form of practice, culturally and economically. In present-day terms, the vocabulary used most frequently to describe this new hybrid is "evidence-based" practice (or medicine), in effect basing the practice on an imagined claim to traditional precepts while borrowing heavily from the principles and methods of the scientific approach.

This blend of traditions does not mean that biomedicine and TKM coexist in complete harmony; if anything, the competition between the two approaches has grown stronger in recent years. Even more so than clinical practice, the emergence of a pharmaceutical industry based on traditional remedies represents a lucrative market with vast potential, meaning that many in South Korea want a share for themselves. This market has also brought controversy to the point of distribution, the pharmacy (*yakkuk*), where the sale of these remedies and related OTC (over-the-counter) products has to be regulated. If these products can be produced according to the appropriate industrial and scientific standards, or so goes the argument, anyone should be able to sell them, taking TKM remedies out of the exclusive control of their practitioners. Not surprisingly, this point has met with considerable resistance from the TKM industry, and today's pharmacy represents a fascinating hybrid of past and present. Moreover, insurance coverage for these remedies and for alternative forms of clinical practice also represents an area of ongoing debate.

In this respect, Dr. Jae-Mo Yang's remarks, which appeared in the introduction, continue to serve as a valuable reminder of the challenges of medical pluralism, even as the South Korean government has consistently promoted its modern image. South Koreans now have an increasingly wide variety of medical options from which to choose, with many mixing the use of biomedicine and other forms of practice, depending on circumstances and perceived need. A close friend, for example, informed me that his wife gave birth to twins in a hospital, with the labor taking a number of hours. After experiencing significant lower back pain, along with discomfort in the waist area, she found that the medication prescribed did not provide relief; she instead chose to undergo acupuncture, which reduced the pain and swelling.[16] This kind of approach, remaining open to alternatives, even in a society where much of medical practice has changed dramatically with professionalization, informs the behavior of many South Koreans.

Equally fascinating is the public discourse concerning "unlicensed practitioners," whereby those holding TKM degrees, having invested time and expense in their training, actively police the boundaries of their own profession.[17] In many cases, the individual in question turns out to be an elderly practitioner who began working several decades ago, prior to the emergence of new forms of pedagogy. In cases like this, the individual is typically not dealt with harshly, even as the practice has to be curbed or limited. In other cases, particularly with the sale of remedies or preparations, the TKM community is quite vigilant, protecting its claim over both the preparation and the sale of these goods. In effect, TKM practitioners are just as zealous as medical doctors in defending the rigor and scientific character of their work, as well as in creating a lucrative professional space for themselves.

And it is this last point that unites the diverse collection of South Korean medical practitioners, regardless of their education and background, as the medical profession has become one of the most respected and valued. When I first resided in Seoul in the mid-1990s, this was not necessarily the case, especially prior to the 1997 Asian financial crisis, when the appeal of starting a company made for a good deal of experimentation. While I do not want to suggest that Korean undergraduates pursuing medicine do so motivated only by financial concerns, it is not difficult to illustrate the growing popularity of medicine as a career choice within the last two decades and, in particular, the links between this choice and the growth of private practice. Rather than a heavily socialized form of health care, with its coverage distributed as widely as possible, the South Korean health system has moderated its most recent period of expansion dating to the late 1980s and early 1990s (in 1989), the period associated with the transition to democratization. It has quietly become a plural system, not just with respect to embracing TKM, but equally with its heavy reliance on encouraging access to forms of private care.

In adopting this approach, the ROK does not differ significantly from that taken by other large countries, essentially allowing a two-tiered system to develop on the basis of class and region, with those of means holding far more options. What is surprising, though, is how much this reality differs from the typical stories told about South Korea and its prominent role as a developmental model, still a very powerful narrative in the aftermath of the events of 1989 through 1991 throughout much of Eastern Europe. Moreover, the absence of this material reality from public discourse is equally remarkable, as the medical industry has grown enormously powerful and successfully wards off most attempts at establishing further regulation. It is not unusual, for the period following 1997, to see stories about doctors and medical workers going on strike, with this activity carefully coordinated to extract concessions from legislators.

This book does not seek to offer a critique of the South Korean medical system per se but, rather, to illustrate how it arrived at the present moment historically. In contrast to a narrative of "late" arrival in the provision of health care, a common theme in much of the developmental literature, I have sought to show the origins of a pattern, beginning with an initial period of confusion, followed by extensive rehabilitation efforts in the aftermath of the Korean War. With postwar stability came the massive public health campaigns of the 1960s, with a highly mobilized society permitting a corresponding degree of intervention through the nation's civil institutions: local government offices, public schools, and, perhaps most important, the military. If these forms of care were subsidized throughout much of the period by international donors, the visibility of these external partners was probably not that high at the actual point of distribution.

If much of the planning and execution of the FP and antiparasite campaigns was marked by a top-down style of practice, this does not mean that there was not sufficient room to accommodate the ambitions of individual South Korean citizens. In fact, this was one of the brilliant selling points throughout much of this period, tying the individual's well-being to intertwined themes of personal and national betterment. A healthier population, equipped with the skills to live longer, would also tend to work more longer and more efficiently in new positions, be willing to migrate and live in new types of spaces, and sacrifice for the sake of the next generation, with the family unit standing in for the nation. In a very real sense, the mobilization of biomedicine has led to a very different kind of Korean family; specifically, a much smaller unit, living in an apartment more frequently than not and maintaining a high degree of mobility. These trends reflect not only the fulfillment of the desires of successive South Korean governments but, equally, longer patterns of cultural changes dating to the late colonial period.

Military and Medical Modernity: "Emergency" or Crisis Medicine

When I began this project nearly a decade ago in 2004, I expected to find significant rupture with colonial forms of practice, given the theme of rejection present in much of the Korean historiography. Indeed, South Korea is a very different place than it was in 1948, and its medical system provides a relatively high standard of care, even as access to that care remains very much in question. The high degree of continuity for the period dominated by military rule (from 1948 through 1987) has less to do with the wholesale adoption of Japanese models of practice, arguably, and more to do with the means of its execution—a brute efficiency and the willingness to carry out successive mobilizations at the national scale. Reaching out through its major civil institutions—hospitals, clinics, schools, and the military—and a wide variety of media, the ROK government achieved a level of saturation that made it extremely difficult to evade its message.

Along with the areas covered in the six chapters of this book, there remain numerous subjects that could be referred to only in passing and that deserve greater coverage in a subsequent project. For the military, specifically, its emphasis on reproductive education for home reserve forces at the decommissioning stage, mentioned in Chapter 4, represents one of the ongoing legacies of family planning. Indeed, there is hardly a South Korean male who does not know of the lectures regarding voluntary sterilization (vasectomy), whether through personal experience or conveyed by anecdote, as the practice has been discontinued. Military psychiatry is another such area, an absolutely vital part of maintaining discipline within the armed forces in a country that has participated in two major conflicts and that has maintained its tense border with North Korea for nearly sixty years (from 1953 to the present).

This last remark carries implications for the autopsy, which, although it has been referred to in several places, deserves even greater attention as a stand-alone topic. Even as South Koreans have become far more comfortable with the clinical research culture of biomedicine, the necessity of intervening in both life and death, much of this process was framed until recently within a militarized culture whereby the results of an inquiry remained subject to the whims of political circumstances. With the work performed on "truth and reconciliation" in the past decade, for example, it is now easy to find numerous case records of suspicious deaths, with individuals dying under unusual circumstances, whether from a bump on the head or perhaps even murkier causes. One has to speculate, particularly for the late Park years through the late 1980s (from 1972 through 1987), about how the culture of medicine was shaped—and perhaps even severely distorted—by successive South Korean military regimes, with medical pathologists knowing that it might be better not to examine too closely.

Ultimately, South Korea has successfully transformed itself, and these concluding remarks should take nothing away from the nation's many accomplishments. But if we look at the history closely, rather than as a progressive narrative of democratization and greater access to health care, the material reality here approximates a narrative of state-sanctioned violence in the form of bodily intervention, with the combined potential of an ambitious social science and an aggressive biomedicine reaching directly into South Korean offices, homes, and villages. There were still spaces to circumvent some of this activity; indeed, we have seen a variety of forms of resistance—some even comical—but, in the end, the ROK state has successfully performed the disruptive work of internal colonization on much of its domestic population over a period of three to four decades, leaving rural villagers (the "traditional") behind for a new type of favored citizen: an ideal much cleaner, healthier, and disciplined. This history of class-based violent encounter needs to be recovered, both so as not to repeat the same mistakes in the domestic sphere and also so as not to mobilize it as a model for other developing nations internationally, including North Korea, whatever may happen to that unfortunate nation in the future.

Reference Matter

Notes

Introduction

1. Yang, "A Comprehensive Study," 1960, 71–76.

2. *Ibid.*, 71.

3. *Ibid.*, 71.

4. *Ibid.*, 73.

5. *Ibid.*, 75.

6. Truman, Inaugural Address.

7. Brazinsky, *Nation-Building in South Korea.*

8. DiMoia, "Atoms for Sale?" 589–618.

9. Chemical fertilizer would be an imported item until the early 1960s and would experience shortages until the early 1970s.

10. "Free World," a USIS (U.S. Information Service) publication, popularized this language in South Korea.

11. Klein, *Cold War Orientalism.*

12. While MASH (Mobile Army Surgical Hospital) is probably familiar to many Americans, NORMASH, its Norwegian equivalent, would also play a significant role, carrying over into post–Korean War medical relief.

13. Hughes, "Arterial Repair," 555–561.

14. Seth, *Education Fever.*

15. Suh, "Korean Medicine between the Local and the Universal."

16. Park, *Corporeal Colonialism.*

17. For the longer history of medicine in late Chosŏn and colonial Korea (1876–1910, 1910–1945), see the work of Korean scholars, especially the publications of Park Yunjae of Kyunghee University and Shin Dong-Won of KAIST.

18. Suh, "Korean Medicine between the Local and the Universal."

19. Balfour et al., "Korea," *Public Health and Demography in the Far East*, 61–70.

20. Holt with Wisner, *The Seed from the East*; Oh, "Into the Arms of America."

21. In the Oh dissertation (2008), see chapter 3 regarding "Christian Americanism" and the adoption of Korean "GI babies." See also Eleana Kim, *Adopted Territory*.

22. Rusk, *A World to Care For*.

23. Kim, "Contesting Bodies."

24. Rogaski, *Hygienic Modernity*.

25. The Chamsil apartments, built in southeast Seoul in the mid-1970s, are one example. The reserve training incentives and lectures began in 1971.

26. Wong, *Healthy Democracies*.

27. *The National Medical Center in Korea*.

Chapter 1

1. Grajdanzev, *Modern Korea*.

2. Licensing and Registration Certificate. Byun Sang-hun (1902–1989) continued the practice started by his grandfather, Byun Seok-hong (1846–1926), and father, Byun Yeong-mok (1878–1923), in 1902. The current Dr. Byun, Byun Kil-Won, represents the fifth generation of medical practitioners in the family. See "A Modern Doctor."

3. The USAMGIK, or U.S. Army Military Government in Korea, represented the occupying authority on the southern half of the peninsula from September 1945 to August 1948, with its powers gradually transferred to a provisional government beginning in 1947. See "Liberation and War" (1945–1960) in *Pictorial History of Modern Medicine in Korea*.

4. Licensing and Registration Certificate.

5. *Seoul Taehakkyo Ŭikwahaksa Charyojip* I contains the terms of Allen's agreement with the Korean government. See also Park et al., *Chaedong Chejungwŏn ŭi kyumo wa hwaktae Kwajŏng*, pp. 29–53, for a discussion of the design and function of Allen's hospital site, and Park's *Jejoongwon* for the Allen story.

6. Resumé (*iryŏksŏ*) and Self-Introduction. The term *ŭisaeng*, assigned to traditional practitioners beginning with the 1913 licensing regulation instituted by Japan, implies a trainee or student of lesser status, in contrast to those trained in Western medicine.

7. The CATS sites (Civil Affairs Training Schools), based at university sites distributed throughout the United States, offered language and culture-specific training (during the years 1942 to 1945) to American military personnel preparing for the projected occupations of Europe (Italy, Germany) and Japan. See Leeke, *When Americans Came to Korea*, for an account of an American officer who underwent this training at Stanford before serving in Korea. Also see *Records of the School of Military Government, 1943–1945*.

8. Robertson (Suh), "Legacy of Empire."

9. SKIG (South Korean Interim Government) would assume a portion of the governing functions by 1947.

10. Lada, Chapter XVI, "Philippines and Okinawa."

11. Turner, "Chapter XVIII: Japan and Korea," pp. 659–707.

12. While there is a rich literature in English regarding the occupations of Germany and Japan, Austria and Korea have received far less scholarly attention. For Austria, see Carafano, *Waltzing into the Cold War*; for Korea, see Meade, *American Military Government in Korea*.

13. The original USAMGIK projection had called for the transfer of these positions to Korean hands by January 1946.

14. Shin, "*Kunjŏnggi ŭi Pogŏn Ŭiryo Chŏngch'aek*," pp. 212–232.

15. "Typhus, Small Pox Control Health Bureau's Big Task, RG 554, Box 20, Public Health & Welfare, Health of Troops." Also see "Misc. Typed Materials," Public Health & Welfare, RG 554, Box 19.

16. Underwood, "Education in Korea."

17. Turner, "Chapter XVIII: Japan and Korea," p. 692. According to Turner, USAMGIK estimated that about 30 percent of the trained physicians resided in Seoul, administering to only about 5 percent of the population.

18. Schmid, *Korea between Empires, 1885–1919*. See especially chapters 1 and 2, "Decentering the Middle Kingdom and Realigning the East" and "Engaging a Civilizing Japan," for the Korean court's changing attitude toward Chinese culture in its official discourse at the end of the nineteenth century.

19. *Activities of Severance Union Medical College and Severance Hospital, 1927–28*.

20. Don Baker offers one of the best surveys of TKM in "Oriental Medicine in Korea," in Sellin (ed.), *Medicine across Cultures*, pp. 133–154. Son provides one of the few surveys covering all three periods: "Modernization of Medical Care in Korea, 1876–1990." Han's "The Rise of Western Medicine and Revival of Traditional Medicine in Korea: A Brief History" looks primarily at the return of interest in traditional medicine corresponding with recent economic growth in the 1980s. See also Kim, "In the Margins: Writing on Medicine in Korea after 1876."

21. See Baker, pp. 150–152.

22. I am referring here in to a number of MPhil and DPhil theses that have emerged from Cambridge University and the Needham Research Institute: Andrews, "The Making of Modern Chinese Medicine, 1895–1937"; Taylor, "The History of the Barefoot Doctors" and "Medicine of Revolution"; Smith, "To Revise and to Improve."

23. See Sellin 2003.

24. Kim, "Hybrid Modernity."

25. It should not be surprising that Japanese soldiers, who may have had access to *kampo* (Chinese medicine in Japan) at home would seek similar remedies in this new setting.

26. Dr. Byun Kil-Won, interviews, June 16 and 25, 2006.

27. *Ibid.* Korea is a culture with a long tradition of documents, certainly, but personal diaries or similar types of materials were far less common during Japanese colonialism and the early ROK.

28. "Official accounts" include Japanese colonial surveys, USAMGIK Bureau of Public Health & Welfare surveys (the Smith Report), and estimates provided by the ROK public health bureau.

29. Baker, "Oriental Medicine in Korea."

30. *Ibid.*

31. Dr. Byun Kil-Won, interviews, June 16 and 25, 2006. While the family does not maintain a log of patients for this period, Byun Sang-hun's personal prescriptions have been kept via his handwritten annotations to his personal library of medical texts.

32. The end of the royal examination system, along with the training of local physicians in biomedicine, signaled the marginalization of traditional practice within the Korean court (Baker, p. 152). According to the Byun family, Byun Seok-hong was specifically asked by King Kojong to serve the residents of central Korea.

33. Underwood, *Korea in War, Revolution and Peace.* Underwood's title at SNU was *kyomuch'ŏjang*, which translates as director of academic affairs. In his memoir, Underwood describes the position as analogous to that of a university registrar. Interviews with Horace G. Underwood, January 10 and 13 and February 13, 2003.

34. Clark, *Living Dangerously in Korea.* See also Underwood, *Challenged Identities*, and Kim, "Christianity in Colonial Korea."

35. Moon and Kim, *Han'guk Kŭndae Kwahak Hyŏngsŏng Kwajŏng Charyo*. See also Kim, "The Growth of Scientific-Technological Manpower during the Japanese Colonial Period"; Dr. Kim's thesis is also available in an updated version published in 2005.

36. Clark, *Living Dangerously in Korea.*

37. Underwood, *Korea in War, Revolution and Peace.*

38. Smith Report, "Some Problems in Public Health in Korea."

39. Baker, "Oriental Medicine in Korea," p. 148. See also Shin, "The License System for Korean Herbal Practitioners in 1900."

40. Shin, "The License System," p. 481.

41. Baker, "Oriental Medicine in Korea," pp. 139–140.

42. *Ibid.*

43. *Ibid.*

44. *Ibid.*

45. *Ibid.*

46. The June 1999 issue of *Tongbang Hakchi* is devoted almost exclusively to the topic of Korean traditional medicine, focusing in particular on the Chosŏn period.

47. Kim, *Chosŏn Sidae Ŭigwan Sŏnbal*, pp. 1–93.

48. Baker passes over this issue fairly quickly, citing the Han, Sui, and Tang dynasties as "primary sources of [Koryo] medical concepts and practices" (p. 137). To

begin to trace the numerous sources underlying what later became Korean tradition, see Kim, *Han'guk ŭihaksa* and "Middle Eastern and Western Influence on the Development of Korean Medicine."

49. Baker, "Oriental Medicine in Korea," p. 142.

50. *Ibid.*, p. 143.

51. *Ibid.*

52. *Ibid.*, pp. 146–147.

53. Shin, "The License System," p. 480.

54. *Ibid.*, p. 481.

55. At the same time, court physicians were retained in an official capacity through the late nineteenth century, as Baker points out, meaning that the transition was not an abrupt one (Baker, "Oriental Medicine in Korea").

56. Yeo, "Han mal kwa ilche sigi sŏn'gyo ŭisadŭl ŭi chŏnt'ong ŭihak insik kwa yŏn'gu."

57. *Ibid.*

58. *Ibid.*

59. *Ibid.*

60. *Ibid.*

61. *Ibid.*

62. *Ibid.*

63. *Ibid.*

64. *Ibid.*

65. *Ibid.*

66. According to his *iryŏksŏ*, Byun Sang-hun attended a (Japanese) normal school until the age of nineteen, graduating in 1921.

67. It is fair to assume that the family had already begun the process of accommodating to a program of self-study.

68. Byun Kil-won, interviews, June 16 and 25, 2006.

69. The materials of which the needles were composed, as well as the method of placement, would have been influenced by the interaction with biomedicine.

70. These transcribed notes indicate that medical tradition was viewed as a process, rather than a static set of practices.

71. He also became a father in 1925, adding to his responsibilities.

72. Byun's documents indicate that he registered three times under Japanese rule, in 1938, 1941, and 1944 (Byun Family Papers).

73. In the 1930s, the *T'ongsŏ nonjaeng*, or East–West medical controversy, was the subject of numerous editorials and opinion pieces.

74. There are published anthologies of these editorials; see the related project headed by Yeo In-Sok of Severance Hospital at Yonsei University.

75. Sawada, *Cultural Politics in Imperial Japan and Colonial Korea.*

76. *Ibid.*

77. *Sŏul Taehakkyo Ŭigwahaksa Charyojip* covers the transition from government hospital to a Japanese-run facility. See especially pp. 1–40 for the photographic record.

78. *Severance Union Medical College Catalog, 1925–1926.*

79. "Report of the Special Committee of the Faculty of Chosen Christian College."

80. Moon and Kim, *Han'guk kŭndae.*

81. Wells, "The Rationale of Korean Economic Nationalism," pp. 822–859.

82. *Sŏul Taehakkyo Ŭigwahaksa Charyojip, 89.*

83. *Ibid.*

84. *Ibid.*

85. Choo Kun Won, interview, October 20, 2005, SNU Hospital, Alumni Building.

86. Byun Kil-won, interviews, June 16 and 25, 2006.

87. The meetings held during the war years indicate that the local government was interested in using traditional doctors in some fashion.

88. Resumé (*iryŏksŏ*), Byun Family Papers.

89. *Ibid.*

90. The U.S. Strategic Bombing Survey took numerous aerial photographs of Korean industrial sites, primarily in the North, in late 1944.

91. Résumé (*iryŏksŏ*), Byun Family Papers.

92. *Ibid.* Byun does not specify the content of this meeting.

93. Smith Report, "Some Problems in Public Health in Korea," pp. 19–21.

94. *Ibid.*

95. *Ibid.*

96. *Kamsajang*, in the possession of Dr. Byun Kil-Won.

97. See the Conclusion to this book.

Chapter 2

1. Gordin, *Five Days in August*; see especially Chapter 1.

2. Planning for the various postwar scenarios began as early as mid-1942 with the formation of a School for Military Government at the University of Virginia. In addition, a set of civil affairs training schools (CATS) provided language and area-specific training, with many of those destined for Japan and Korea training at Yale University. For the CATS program of pedagogy on public health, see the Records of the Army Specialized Training Division, Yale University, and also the class lectures for CATS and public health contained in the C. E. A. Winslow Papers.

3. Morris-Suzuki, "Invisible Immigrants," pp. 119–153; see also Morris-Suzuki's subsequent book on the topic, *Borderline Japan*.

4. Turner, "Chapter XVIII, Japan and Korea," pp. 691–704; especially see "Medical Influence in Prewar Korea."

5. *Ibid.*, pp. 692–693.

6. *History of Evacuation and Repatriation through the Port of Pusan*, p. 1. See also Yang's *Technology of Empire*.

7. Barry, *The Great Influenza.*

8. *History of Evacuation and Repatriation through the Port of Pusan*, p. 29.

9. *Ibid.*, p. 28.

10. For Willard's brief biography, see *Journal of Medical Education*, December 1972, 851–852, and for a longer account, see West, with Coggins, *A Special Kind of Doctor*, pp. 30–32.

11. Charles Edward Amory Winslow Papers, Yale University; see especially Section IV. Academic Papers, "Yale University Civil Affairs Training School, Section on Public Health." See also Records of the Army Specialized Training Division, Yale University, 1940–1963.

12. *Ibid.*

13. Turner, "Chapter XVIII: Japan and Korea," pp. 689–690.

14. Willard, "Some Problems," pp. 661–670.

15. Willard, *Medical Education and Medical Care in Alabama.*

16. *Ibid.*

17. The Tenth Army was founded in 1944, but it is fair to assume an accumulation of knowledge deriving from earlier Pacific campaigns, as well as the lengthy American experience in the Philippines.

18. Those who had CATS training for Japan often ended up in Korea, on the assumption that their training was close enough to be able to work successfully in this setting. See Leeke, *When Americans Came to Korea*, for an account of an American officer who underwent CATS training at Stanford before serving in Korea. Also see *Records of the School of Military Government, 1943–1945.*

19. "Part V. The Pacific."

20. Park et al., "Chaedong Chejungwŏn ŭi Kyumo wa Hwaktae Kwajŏng," pp. 29–53, for a discussion of the design and function of Horace Allen's original hospital site, and Park's *Jejoongwon* for the Allen story as understood in Korea.

21. An abbreviated account of the story of missionary origins can be found at http://medicine.yonsei.ac.kr/en/About_YUCM/Introduction/.

22. The documents for USAMGIK concerning this outbreak are at NARA, but I rely here on the copies available through the Korean National Archive in Taejeon. See www.koreanhistory.or.kr/.

23. Smith Report, "Some Problems in Public Health in Korea."

24. Suh, "Korean Medicine Between the Local and the Universal." See chapter 2, "Medical Reforms and Institutional Change."

25. *Sŏul Taehakkyo Ŭigwahaksa Charyojip.* For current data on the respective alumni groups (KIU and KMC), there is a CDR available from Dr. Joo Koo Han of SNUH, current to 2004.

26. *Monthly Summary of Nonmilitary Activities in Korea and Japan*, "Student Unrest," p. 65.

27. In more recent NK material on health, the materials, partially reliable, derive from NGOs and the World Health Organization.

28. Park, "Corporeal Colonialism"; see also the work of Sonja Kim (SUNY-Binghamton) on Japanese colonialism and "mothering" policy, Theodore Jun Yoo (University of Hawaii-Manoa) on psychiatry, Jennifer Yum (graduate student, Harvard University) on postwar medicine, Jane Kim (graduate student, UCLA) on leprosy, Suh Soyoung (Dartmouth College) on traditional medicine, and Jennifer Jung Kim (lecturer, UCLA) on gender.

29. This claim reflects material reality—continuity with Japanese models of health practice—and in part a construction, a gesture allowing for the mobilization of reforms.

30. Morris-Suzuki, *Borderline Japan*.

31. The set of rules governing what could be carried was motivated by the question of Japanese reparations, but it is unclear why it held for Koreans returning from Japan.

32. Morris-Suzuki emphasizes this point in *Borderline Japan*, noting that most studies only focus on one country in isolation, typically Japan.

33. Crawford Sams, oral history interview at WUSTL (re 1945–1951).

34. Aldous, "Typhus in Occupied Japan." See also Aldous and Suzuki, *Reforming Public Health in Occupied Japan , 1945–1952*.

35. Morris-Suzuki, "Invisible Immigrants."

36. *Ibid.*

37. Sams, "*Medic*," p. 207.

38. *Ibid.*

39. Willard, "Some Problems," p. 661.

40. *Ibid.*, p. 668.

41. *Ibid.*, p. 666.

42. See the National Archives of Korea at www.koreanhistory.or.kr/ for the USAMGIK "Weekly Military Occupational Activities Report" covering the period from May1946 through January 1947. These reports provide the most detail regarding the perceived cholera outbreak.

43. Pavel Leshakov, Moscow State University, May 2011, personal communication.

44. Millett, *The War for Korea*, p. 50.

45. *Ibid.*

46. *Ibid.*, p. 81.

47. The greatest number of USAMGIK reports covers the months from June through August 1946, with reports on typhus outnumbering those for cholera.

48. Shin and Robinson, *Colonial Modernity*.

49. Henderson, "Human Rights," pp. 125–170. As Henderson notes, the originals are available in *The Ordinances of the U.S. Military Government* (Seoul Official Gazette, Chosŏn Haengjŏng Ch'ulp'ansa, 1946).

50. *Ibid.*

51. *Ibid.* Dr. Kim Nam Il of Kyunghee University maintains some of the original USAMGIK circulars and gazettess and was kind enough to share these materials.

52. Turner, "Chapter XVIII: Japan and Korea," pp. 690 -691; also see p. 705.

53. *Ibid.*

54. Korean National Archives.

55. Turner, "Chapter XVIII: Japan and Korea," p. 696.

56. *Ibid.*

57. *Ibid.*, pp. 706–707.

58. This type of restriction was about limiting mobility: In some cases, roadblocks were set up.

59. The terms of the "Moscow Agreement" were announced late in 1945.

60. Millett, *The War for Korea*, p. 81.

61. Shin, *Hoyŏlcha, Chosŏn ŭl Sŭpkyŏk Hada : Mom kwa Ŭihak ŭi Han'guksa. Sŏul : Yŏksa Pip'yŏngsa*. See also Delaporte, *Disease and Civilization*.

62. Willard, "Some Problems," p. 661.

63. Millet focuses on this a great deal.

64. USAMGIK declared its efforts a success by late 1946.

65. Willard, "Some Problems," p. 663.

66. *Ibid.*

67. *Ibid.*

68. *Ibid.*, p. 664.

69. *Ibid.*, p. 663.

70. *Ibid.*

71. *Ibid.*, p. 666.

72. *Ibid.*, p. 663.

73. Balfour et al., *Public Health and Demography in the Far East*, p. 51.

74. Kim, "Limiting Birth."

75. Balfour et al., *Public Health and Demography in the Far East*, p. 63. See also Cullather, *The Hungry World*, especially chapter 1.

76. *Ibid.*, p. 65.

77. *Ibid.*, p. 68.

78. Fruhstuck, *Colonizing Sex*, p. 109.

79. Balfour et al., *Public Health and Demography in the Far East*, p. 61.

Chapter 3

An earlier version of some of the material covered in this chapter was published in John P. DiMoia. "From Minnesota to Seoul? The DeWall Helix Bubble Oxygenator and Technology Transfer in Open-Heart Surgery, 1955–1965." *Comparative Technology Transfer and Society* 7.2 (2009), pp. 201–225.

1. Lee, "Resection Therapy in Pulmonary Tuberculosis."

2. For the context of medical relief efforts during the Korean War, see the work of the American-Korean Foundation (AKF), Howard A. Rusk Papers, Folder 287, American-Korean Foundation, 1.

3. Yonsei University Severance Hospital.

4. Kim and Hwang, "The Minnesota Project," pp. 112–123. See also Lee, "Minesot'a P'ŭrojekt'ŭ ka Han'guk Ŭihak Kyoyuk e Mich'in Yŏnghyang (The Influence of the Minnesota Project on Korean Medical Education)"; and Gault, "Korea—A New Venture in International Medical Education," pp. 73–85. For cardiovascular surgery at SNU, see *Sŏul Taehakkyo Hyungbu Oegwahak Kyosil*. For a contemporary account of the project, see "How the U Helps Seoul University Rebuild after the Ravages of War." As for the international assistance, a consortium of three Scandinavian nations—Sweden, Norway, and Denmark—assisted in the refurbishment of the National Medical Center (Kungnip Ŭiryowŏn), based at the site of the former Seoul City Hospital. See *The National Medical Center in Korea*.

5. *The Veterans Administration Hospital and The University of Minnesota Medical School; Minneapolis VA (Veterans Administration) Hospital Manual of Standard Procedures*.

6. See RG 286 at National Archives concerning predecessor organizations to USAID from 1949 to 1961).

7. Similar changes in medical pedagogy and surgery were also taking place at Severance Hospital and the National Medical Center.

8. Lee, "Resection Therapy in Pulmonary Tuberculosis." For Dr. Lillehei's story, see Miller, *King of Hearts*.

9. Dr. Lee soon passed along leadership of this activity to younger colleagues.

10. The label "thoracic surgery" was mobilized at the time. The actual practice of perfecting the surgery, however, took considerable time to develop.

11. The University of Minnesota did not have its own thoracic surgery unit until 1965. To offer another comparison, the National Medical Center (NMC) did not allow Korean doctors to develop specialties at this time.

12. Dr. Neil Gault, interview, November 2005.

13. *Sŏul Taehakkyo Ŭigwahaksa Charyojip* p. 89. See also the Keijo Imperial University materials stored at Seoul National University library.

14. Kim, "Physicians on the Move."

15. Je Geun Chi, "Sŏul Taehakkyo Ŭigwa Taehak Pyŏngnihak Kyosil 50-yŏnsa (First 50 Years of Department of Pathology Seoul National University College of Medicine)."

16. These perceptions appear not only in the reports issued on behalf of the Minnesota Project but also in those from the NMC.

17. Yonsei and Severance had first proposed a union after liberation, but the Korean War delayed the move.

18. Kim and Hwang, "The Minnesota Project," p. 120. The National Medical Center was also implementing these new professional categories, with both sites emphasizing clinical practice.

19. The Ninth Meeting of the William T. Peyton Society, Honoring the Contributions of Lyle A. French. Lyle French was largely responsible for starting the neurosurgery program, comparable to the cardiac program. Under his training, Dr. Shim Bo Sung received a Minnesota degree and started a neurosurgery program at Seoul National University Hospital. For Korean accounts, see *Department of Neurosurgery, Seoul National University College of Medicine: 50th Anniversary* (1957–2007) and Kim and Park, Shim Bo-Sung.

20. Dr. Kim Ock-Joo and Takuya Miyagawa of Seoul National University have done research on this topic.

21. Rusk, *A World to Care For.*

22. This story is available through the SNU student newspaper, *Taehak Sinmun.*

23. The United States Information Service (USIS) would publish a publication series titled "Free World," with its Korean version appearing as "*Chayu Segye*," popularizing this label.

24. Harold Stassen and University of Minnesota President James Morrill (1945–1960) also had a personal connection via Stassen's period as the state's governor.

25. Bronfenbrenner, *Academic Encounter*, pp. 170–173.

26. *Taehak Sinmun*, 1950–1954.

27. Bronfenbrenner, *Academic Encounter*, pp. 170–173.

28. Weems, letter of April 3, 1955, to Morrill. See also Staley, "Report on the College of Engineering, Seoul National University," UMN.

29. Weems, letter of April 3, 1955, to Morrill.

30. Maloney, "Report of Observations as Adviser in Medicine"; Flink, "Report and Recommendations on Teaching and Research in Internal Medicine"; Brown, "Report of Observation and Activities as Adviser in Medicine"; Mitchell, "Report on the Seoul National University Hospital"; and Matthews, "Final Report of Observations and Recommendations." In total, eleven Minnesota advisers spent time in Seoul.

31. Schimert, *Final Report of Observations, Activities, and Recommendations Concerning the College of Medicine, Seoul National University.* See also Wangensteen's "Report to Dean Howard's Subcommittee."

32. Surgery Department 1007:33 "Schimert." This file contains the personal letters between Schimert and his UMN superiors (Wangensteen in particular). UMN. See also Schimert, *Final Report.*

33. Smith Report, "Some Problems in Public Health in Korea," p. 89.

34. Hospitals tended to adopt a triage approach, admitting only those patients likely to fare well.

35. There would be many points of contact, but especially with the United States and Europe.

36. Lillehei et al., "Direct Vision Intracardiac Surgery in Man ," pp. 1–8.

37. Hence the term *blue baby* for a child with oxygen deficiency.

38. DeWall, *The Helix Reservoir Bubble Oxygenator for Use in Open Intracardiac Surgery.* See DeWall, "Introduction to the Problem," p. 10.

39. "Heart Refrigeration Operation—Lewis." UMN.

40. This apocryphal story appears in *King of Hearts*, but I have been unable to trace it back any further. Miller, *King of Hearts*, p. 84.

41. Sigmamotor, Inc. Retrieved on November 12, 2012, from http://sigmamotorinc.com/history_sigma_motor.html.

42. *Ibid.*

43. DeWall does not mention these considerations in his thesis, as he was still thinking in terms of resolving the situation at UMN Hospital. DeWall also does not mention the story regarding beer bubbles, which appears only in Miller. The issue of transportability would become critical as the number of international residents at Minnesota began to increase.

44. This would mean increasing print coverage, and it intersected nicely with the postwar arrival of television.

45. Dr. George Schimert, Curriculum Vitae. An earlier version of the CV is in Schimert's personnel file at University of Minnesota Hospital.

46. "They Appreciate Dogs That Died."

47. Lee, letter of August 30, 1965, to Lillehei, p. 1.

48. Minnesota would send a total of eleven advisers to Seoul between 1954 and 1962.

49. Schimert had only been in the United States a few years (having migrated from Germany) and was very eager to further his career.

50. Schimert's personnel file at the UMN Hospital contains numerous references to these doubts, but unfortunately the contents of the file may not be cited without permission from his wife, Florence Schimert.

51. Wangensteen, letter to Schimert, February 3, 1958.

52. Schimert, "Chest Surgery," *Final Report*, p. 13.

53. Diehl, letter to Schimert, January 27, 1958. This letter also contains Wangensteen's handwritten comments supporting Diehl's view.

54. *Ibid.*

55. Wangensteen, letter to Paine, April 27, 1960, 2. "Schimert."

56. George Schimert, "A Simple Bubble Type of Pump-Oxygenator for Intracardiac Surgery."

57. Kim Ok-Joo points out that, by the project's completion, of the more than 100 SNU staff members at the hospital, more than 80 percent had studied abroad, seventy-seven at Minnesota.

58. Schimert, "Chest Surgery," *Final Report*, p. 13.

59. Schimert, "A Review of the Present State of Intracardiac Surgery," pp. 68–73.

60. In other words, there was a great deal of prior work leading up to the 1956 publications.

61. "Townspeople Send Girl, 3, Here for Surgery."

62. "Conquest" Reports on Miraculous New Heart Surgery, March 9, 1955. CBS.

63. This was a claim made by Minnesota, not by the Koreans.

64. Schimert does not single the open-heart case in his report, although it clearly assumed greater significance for him later in life, when he would try to claim priority for performing the "first" open-heart procedure in Asia. Lee Young-Gyun does write of it, however, in a postcard to Lillehei dated August 24, 1959, briefly describing both the case (a VSD) and result—"several hours survival"—to his mentor. Lee, letter of August 24, 1959. See also Kaleida Health at www.kaleidahealth.org/news/archive/1200/121200.asp.

65. The series of letters to Lillehei would continue until his death.

66. Lee Young-Gyun's publications indicate that he worked with a number of different surgical partners.

67. The Korean team created a dog service, working with animals when no human subjects were available.

68. Dr. Chu Jeong-hwa, interview.

69. *Ibid.*

70. Lee Young-Gyun, personal and surgical records.

71. *Ibid.*

72. *Ibid.*

73. *Ibid.*

74. Dr. Lee, letter of August 30, 1965, to Lillehei.

75. Dr. Kim Won-Gon, personal communication. Interview with NMC museum staff (December 2010).

76. Lee, letter of February 27, 1959.

77. *Ibid.*

78. *Ibid.*, 2.

79. *Ibid.*, 1.

80. *Ibid.*

81. *Ibid.*, p .2.

82. *Ibid.*

83. Lee, letter of June 8, 1961, to Lillehei.

84. *Ibid.*

85. From the late 1950s, Lillehei's team received national publicity.

86. Lee, letter of June 8, 1961, to Lillehei.

87. *Ibid.*

88. SigmaMotor; retrieved on November 12, 2012, from http://sigmamotorinc.com/history_sigma_motor.html.

89. *Ibid.*

90. *PVC ŭi Kasoje. Anjŏngje e Kwanhan Yŏn'gu.*

91. Lee, letter of July 1, 1963, to Lillehei.

92. Lee, letter of July 22, 1961, to Lillehei.

93. Heparin's clinical use dates to the mid-1930s.

94. See *The Journal of Comparative Technology Transfer* (JHU).

95. At about this time, North Korea appealed increasingly to its own version of traditional medicine.

96. Lee, letter of May 14, 1963, to Lillehei.

97. *Ibid.*

98. Lee, letter of August 30, 1965, to Lillehei.

99. The United States seems highly likely, given 1965 changes to immigration law.

100. Lee, *Developmental Dictatorship.*

101. Dr. Lee would experience short-term surgical success in 1964.

102. Lee, letter of August 30, 1965, to Lillehei, pp. 1–3.

103. *Ibid.*, p. 1.

104. *Ibid.*

105. *Ibid.*

106. This facility was the site of the former Seoul City Hospital.

107. Cooper, *Open Heart: The Radical Surgeons Who Revolutionized Medicine.*

108. *Ibid.*

109. *Ibid.*

110. *Ibid.*

111. Lee, letter of July 2, 1968, to Lillehei.

112. *Ibid.*

113. *Ibid.*

114. *Ibid.*

115. The OR staff went from a single surgeon and one or two assistants to a full surgical team.

116. Kim Tae-ho, personal communication, SNUH, February, 2012

Chapter 4

An earlier version of some of the material covered in this chapter was published in John P. Dimoia, "'Let's Have the Proper Number of Children and Raise Them Well!' Family Planning and Nation-Building in South Korea, 1961–1968." *East Asian Science, Technology and Society*, 2.3, pp. 361–379. Copyright 2008, National Science Council, Taiwan. All rights reserved. Reprinted by permission of the present publisher, Duke University Press.

1. "Mobile Service, 1966."

2. "Korea, Family Planning Program—Historical Review." See also *Pae, Ŭn-gyŏng, Han'guk Sahoe Ch'ulsan Chojŏl ŭi Yŏksajŏk Kwajŏng kwa Chendŏ.*

3. Population Council. Retrieved on September 22, 2011, from www.popcouncil.org/who/history.asp.

4. Hartman, "Korea: Medical Referral System and Mobile Services."

5. Hartman passed away on September 29, 1968, due to a heart attack while working for the South Korean FP program (from 1958 to 1968); "Paul P. Hartman, 1911–1968." See also Certificate of voluntary status for Paul Hartman, "Equipment, 1964–1966." The same box contains a memo, "Possible Employment of Mr. Paul Hartman as a Health Educator for Assignment to Korea."

6. *Ibid.* Prior to his work in Korea, Hartman worked in health education in Illinois, following graduate training at the University of Michigan.

7. "Operation of Mobile Clinics Big Success," WHMC, 8. These operations targeted leprosy.

8. Dr. Sook Bang did graduate work at Michigan and returned to work alongside Dr. Jae-Mo Yang. Frequent contact with American programs like those at Michigan (PSC) and Princeton (OPR) allowed South Korea to accumulate expertise.

9. Freedman, *Observing Taiwan's Demographic Transition.*

10. "Sungdong Project." Re "Seong-dong": The romanization here is not always consistent. See also *Kich'o ŭihak kwa na ŭi sam.* I had the opportunity to interview Dr. Kwon in Seoul, July 2010, with Dr. Kim Ock-Joo of SNUH.

11. PPFK, *The 10(ten)-year History of Family Planning in Korea.*

12. *Ibid.* Andrei Lankov also has a section on the FP slogans in his *The Dawn of Modern Korea.* The section is titled "Three-Three-Thirty-Five," referring to the famous campaign in which women were asked to have a maximum of three children, with the births spaced at three-year intervals, and to stop at thirty-five years of age.

13. "Swedish Development Assistance in the Field of Family Planning, 1969."

14. It is easy to find similar slogans across the national FP programs, providing justification for this claim.

15. Connelly, *Fatal Misconception.*

16. The Taiwan program often used Japanese language in interacting with rural villagers, although I have yet to come across an explicit claim in the Korean context. See note 19, below.

17. Freedman, *Observing Taiwan's Demographic Transition.*

18. Kirk, letter of November 30, 1961, to Takeshita.

19. *Ibid.* Kirk's letter indicates that the Michigan team was well aware of the utility of using Japanese in Taiwan and wanted to use the language in its activities but remained sensitive to the likelihood of encountering "difficulty . . . at the higher echelons," p. 2. See also Minoru Tachi, letter of August 26, 1963, to Marshall Balfour.

Tachi, director of the Institute of Population Problems in Japan (Ministry of Health and Social Welfare), implies that he would not mind contact with the Korean FP program but also emphasizes the official position of the Japanese government, which in 1963 "does not find it in the position of extending assistance."

20. "Korea, Family Planning Program—Historical Review."

21. Kim, "Contesting Bodies"; see especially chapters 3 and 4.

22. "Korea, Family Planning Program—Historical Review."

23. "How to Insert an Intrauterine Loop."

24. Organization of Family Planning Services, Korea. With this kind of centralized system, the FP program was (at least in theory) in contact with every administrative level, down to the tiniest village.

25. Freedman and Takeshita, with contributions by L. P. Chow [and others], *Family Planning in Taiwan.*

26. Bang, Lee, and Yang, "A Survey of Fertility and Attitude toward Family Planning in Rural Korea."

27. The dates/months cited in the article are inconsistent, but 1962 should be a reliable start date, prior to the 1964 national mobilization.

28. Bang, Lee, and Yang, "A Survey of Fertility and Attitude toward Family Planning in Rural Korea."

29. *Ibid.* The Koyang study refers to "non-clinical methods" adopted by villagers, presumably an oblique reference to abortion and other methods that FP would aim to replace; p. 100. Many abortion studies would be published from 1964 to 1967, during the course of the FP program.

30. "TV spot announcement (radio spot announcement and newspaper ad." In addition to advertising on television, on radio, and in print, PPFK also sponsored public exhibitions.

31. Bang, Lee, and Yang, "A Survey of Fertility and Attitude toward Family Planning in Rural Korea," p. 100.

32. *Ibid.*

33. "Chubu ka toemyŏn nuguna" and "namp'yŏn i toemyŏn nuguna" ("Every housewife would like to/Every husband would like to").

34. Kwon, *Ten Years of Urban Population Studies in Korea.*

35. With its reach extending through the different administrative units (To, Kun, Myŏn), the FP bureaucracy claimed that its reach could approach even the smallest village.

36. "Acceptor" was first used as a social science term and appears frequently in the Michigan KAP documents before it was picked up by national programs.

37. "Organizational Report, April 1961–June 1963," p. 1. See also Takeshita, *The Global Biopolitics of the IUD.*

38. Fruhstuck, *Colonizing Sex*, p. 109.

39. "How to Insert an Intrauterine Loop." This is taken from the Rockefeller materials for Taiwan, not South Korea, but it indicates that trainees would have been familiar with the problems associated with insertion.

40. The studies associated with the Seongdong-gu Action Plan specifically would continue well into the 1970s. See also "Sung-dong Project: Key People."

41. "Background: Need for an Action Plan," pp. 9–10. At the beginning of the Korean program, the "menu" held four items: foam tablets, (spermicidal) jelly, the condom, and the loop.

42. "Organizational Report, April 1961–June 1963," p. 1.

43. "Sung-dong Project Substations."

44. Introduced in the late 1920s, this was the model on which Ota based his work.

45. Most estimates for the loop assume about a 25 percent expulsion rate due to a variety of factors.

46. There were no formal clinical trials yet; I mean that this activity approximated what would later become the clinical trial.

47. It was more typical than not to have a trainee do the insertion procedure.

48. As we will see shortly, the insertion was actually quite difficult. "Sung-dong Project: Key People."

49. "Sung-dong Project Substations."

50. *Ibid.*

51. *Ibid.*

52. "Training of Personnel," p. 1.

53. *Ibid.*

54. "Background: Need for an Action Plan," 16.

55. "Loop Production Problem," p. 1.

56. *Ibid.*

57. *Ibid.*, p. 3.

58. "Mr. Hill and Loop Experts," p. 1.

59. *Ibid.*

60. "Family Planning and Workers Creed," p. 1.

61. *Ibid.*

62. *Ibid.*

63. *Ibid.*

64. *Ibid.*

65. "Steps in Inserting the Lippes Loop."

66. "Medical Conditions in Korea."

67. *Ibid.*

68. The program would now have to create a new category to accommodate "reacceptors."

69. Indeed, the vasectomy story receives little mention in the FP historiography for South Korea, although it would form a critical part of reserve army training after 1971.

70. This study covers Seoul and does not show a high degree of class tension, compared with studies of rural areas.

71. Keeny, letter to Hartman, November 25, 1965.

72. *Ibid.*

73. *Ibid.*

74. Letter from Ljunggren to Belsky, p. 1.

75. *Ibid.*

76. *Ibid.*, p. 2.

77. *Ibid.*, p. 3.

78. Lee Hee Yong, "Studies on Vasectomy, 3: Clinical Studies on the Influences of Vasectomy." I am drawing here from across the range of Dr. Lee's late 1960s publications.

79. *Ibid.*

80. The goal of 20,000 a year would never be satisfactorily achieved.

81. As noted earlier, the vasectomy would only reach greater numbers when incorporated as a regular part of military life in the 1970s.

82. Vasectomy poster in the possession of Dr. Kim Nam-Il, Kyunghee University. The bold text reads: "What every man needs to know about these days/today."

83. This holds primarily for urban areas like Seoul, not necessarily for rural areas.

84. Dr. Lee would continue his work well into the following decade.

85. Much of Korean medical care would be heavily subsidized through at least the early 1980s.

86. PPFK, *10-Year History.*

87. *Ibid.*

88. *Ibid.*

89. *Ibid.*

90. *Ibid.*

91. The home reserve started in 1968 as tensions grew with North Korea.

92. Sung, "Evaluation of Population Education Program."

93. The gap between the "K" and the "P" would always present something of a problem.

94. "Preliminary Report of the Joint Kyunggi-Yonsei Family Planning Project (April 1968–March 1970)." Also see the appendix to this report.

95. Sonja Kim traces these groups back to the pre–Korean War period.

96. "Preliminary Report of the Joint Kyunggi-Yonsei Family Planning Project," appendix.

97. This has to remain speculative, but both Japan and Sweden were very interested in contributing materials.

98. "Swedish Grant to Family Planning Programme of the Republic of Korea."

99. PPFK, *10-Year History.*

100. *Ibid.*

101. *Ibid.*

102. For context to the New Village Movement, see the Harvard series, *Studies in the Modernization of the Republic of Korea, 1945–1975*.

103. Mother's Clubs were essentially economic collectives, so FP was only one part of the agenda.

104. "Summary of Field Observation of Kyunggi-Yonsei Family Planning Project."

105. *Ibid.*

106. As many of the actors in family planning were women (midwives, mother's clubs), this should not be surprising. The act of self-reporting to social scientists was new, however.

107. Changing the preference for male children was a major part of the international family planning effort.

108. PPFK. *10-Year History.*

109. *Ibid.*

110. *Ibid.*

111. This figure was created to correspond to the number of villages at the smallest level.

112. The Yushin period of rule would begin in October 1972. These statistics were probably less about state scrutiny of residents than the ability of the ROK government to create a convincing portrait to its international partners.

113. I have received the question about potential male violence at many talks, but PPFK does not document much of this kind of activity. Interviews might yield a different story.

Chapter 5

The author would like to thank Seoul National University (International Summer Institute, 2010) and Kyujanggak Archive for research assistance. In addition, research for Chapter 5 was conducted as part of the "Asian Biopoleis: Biotechnology and Biomedicine as Emergent Forms of Life and Practice" Project, funded by the Ministry of Education, Singapore, and the Humanities and Social Sciences (HSS) Division of the Office of the Deputy President (Research and Technology) at the National University of Singapore (NUS). The period 1969–1995 refers specifically to the school-based campaigns.

1. Hong et al., "A Successful Experience." See also *Paeumyŏ Karŭch'imyŏ* (40th annual volume, SNU Department of Parsitology and Tropical Medicine, and the 50th anniversary volume, *Kisaengch'unghak Kyosil 50-yŏnsa* 2004). Also, see interviews with Hong Sung-Tae, July and December 2010. For the poster, thanks to the Han'guk Kŏn'gang Kwalli Hyŏphoe (Korea Association for Health Promotion, KAHP) and to Dr. Tae-ho Kim of Seoul National University Hospital (SNUH) for assistance in locating a copy of this image. Prior to KAHP, the organization held the name KAPE,

or Korea Association for the Eradication of Parasites. See also *Han'guk Haksaeng Hoech'ung Kamyŏm Chiptan Kwalli Saŏp Punsŏk: Hoech'ung 10-yŏnsa 1969–78.*

2. A literal translation of this text reads, "My health, I find it/search for it."

3. Yonsei University Health System. Retrieved on September 22, 2011, from http://yuhs.iseverance.com/en/about_yuhs/yuhs/YUMC_history/index.asp. We should include leprosy (*nabyŏng*) in this list of common disease problems dating to the post–Korean War era.

4. DiMoia, "Almatke naasŏ hullyunghage kirŭja! (Let's Have the Proper Number of Children and Raise Them Well!)."

5. The majority of these initiatives would share their origins with prewar Japanese colonial efforts at introducing public health on the Korean peninsula. See Kim, "Limiting Birth." See also Kim's PhD thesis, "Contesting Bodies." For the legacy of colonial-era Japan with respect to chronic disease, see the work of Dr. Yunjae Park of Yonsei University.

6. While this was a traditional method, it became necessary after the division of the two Koreas (1945) because heavy industry, including the production of fertilizer, was located in the North. The construction of a urea fertilizer plant at Ch'ungju (Ch'ungju piryo kongjang) (1954–1963) by McGraw-Hydrocarbon began to alleviate the problem, but South Korea did not have its own viable domestic petrochemical industry until at least the early 1970s.

7. Hong et al., "A Successful Experience," p. 179.

8. Baldwin, Jones, and Jones, *America's Rented Troops.*

9. Hartman, "Korea: Medical Referral System and Mobile Services," pp. 10–12.

10. Instruction booklets demonstrating the insertion procedure (in Korean and in English) can be found at the Rockefeller Archive Center (RAC). For more details on training, see "Training of Personnel."

11. OTCA (Overseas Technical Cooperation Agency), annual reports for the years 1966–1970.

12. I refer specifically to the career of Dr. Harujiro Kobayashi for parasitology and Dr. Shiga Kiyoshi for enteric disease.

13. OTCA Annual Reports, 1966–1970.

14. *Ibid.*

15. *Department of Parasitology and Tropical Medicine since 1954.* For the argument about the possible links between reproduction and subsequent biological work in South Korea, see DiMoia, "Almatke naasŏ hullyunghage kirŭja! (Let's Have the Proper Number of Children and Raise Them Well!)." See also Leem and Jin Hee Park, "Rethinking Women and Their Bodies in the Age of Biotechnology," pp. 9–26.

16. I wish to emphasize the developmental context of the Korean life sciences, if not arguing for a direct connection.

17. See Wong, *Betting on Biotech.*

18. In addition to the work of Kobayashi, see the *Keijo Medical Journal*, especially for the late 1930s.

19. Dr. John Arnold, interview, UMN, November 2005.

20. Similarly, Korea has had numerous antirat campaigns.

21. While focused on rats, this campaign fit with the theme of anticorruption.

22. *Seoul through Pictures, Volume 4: Seoul, To Rise Again*, "Public Health and Hygiene," pp. 418 and following.

23. Cho, "Parasitology in a Quickly Changing Society," p. 1.

24. *Ibid*., 2.

25. *Ibid*., 5.

26. Gault, "Observations and Comments on the Seoul National University College of Medicine," pp. 80–81.

27. Kato, *Introduction of a Thick Smear Technique.*

28. *Ibid.*

29. "Birth Control Families to Get Apartment Priority."

30. Moon, *Militarized Modernity.*

31. *Ibid*.; see also Brazinsky, *Nation-Building in South Korea*.

32. Rim, "The Incidence of Intestinal Parasites in ROK Army Soldiers."

33. Along with South Korean troops, Hyundai Construction sent large numbers of its workers to provide logistical support, helping to build airstrips and to dredge in port areas in Thailand and Vietnam. See *The 30 Year History of Hyundai Construction*.

34. South Korea has long had an endemic malaria issue, but it is now considered largely under control. For the problem in Vietnam, see Lee et al., "The Clinical Study of 157 Cases of Malaria Evacuated from Vietnam," pp. 318–326. For American perceptions concerning malaria in Korea, see Hunter, "Local Health Hazards among US Troops Returning from Korea." Hunter would later become famous for his *Hunter's Tropical Medicine*, still in print.

35. Brazinsky, *Nation-Building in South Korea*, pp. 138–140.

36. *Seoul through Pictures, Volume 4, Seoul , To Rise Again*, 1961–1970, p. 57.

37. Kim, "A Socio-Medical Study in Vietnamese Rural Area," pp. 57–70.

38. Kim et al., "Parasitogical Studies of Korean Forces in South Vietnam, II," p. 31.

39. Seo and Rim, "A Study of Malaria amongst Narcotic Addicts in Seoul," pp. 213–220.

40. See bibliography in Seo et al.,"Parasitiological Studies of Korean Forces in South Vietnam, I," p. 28.

41. *Ibid*. The Kato technique was developed for field use, and Seo implies that the Koreans have their own lab resources available for more sophisticated forms of analysis.

42. Kim et al., "Parasitogical Studies of Korean Forces in South Vietnam, II," p. 34.

43. *Ibid*., p. 32.

44. Yang, "A Comprehensive Study of the Health Needs."

45. Lee et al.,"Santonin-Kainic Acid Complex," pp. 79–85.

46. Hong, "Successful Experience," p. 183.

47. *Prevalence of Intestinal Parasitic Infections in Korea*, the 3rd and 4th reports, 1981, 1985 surveys, SNUH library.

Chapter 6

1. Millard, "Oriental Peregrinations," p. 319.

2. Millard, *Cleft Craft*.

3. Gilles and D. R. Millard Jr., *The Principles and Art of Plastic Surgery*. For an earlier context, see Linker, *War's Waste*.

4. Millard, *Saving Faces*.

5. Millard, "Oriental Peregrinations," p. 319.

6. *Ibid*., p. 323.

7. *Ibid*.

8. Napalm was used extensively in the Korean theater, and Millard observes his encounters with burn victims.

9. Millard, "Oriental Peregrinations," p. 328.

10. President Truman integrated the American military after World War II, in 1948.

11. Palumbio-Liu, *Asian/American: Historical Crossings of a Racial Frontier*. See especially pp. 95–104 for a critique of Millard.

12. Millard, "Oriental Peregrinations," p. 334.

13. *Ibid*.

14. *Ibid*. This style of conversion narrative mirrors many of the stories of Korean adoptees.

15. *Ibid*.

16. Millard would also do work with rhinoplasty in the Miami area upon returning to the United States, meaning that he also used the nose as a site of personal and ethnic transformation.

17. Millard, "Oriental Peregrinations," p. 334.

18. *Ibid*.

19. *Ibid*., p. 336.

20. Rusk, *A World to Care For*, p. 142. See also Records of the NYU Medical Center.

21. *Ibid*.

22. *Ibid*., p. 200.

23. *Ibid*., p. 177.

24. Rusk Papers, Folder 287, p. 1.

25. Rusk Papers, Folder 288, p. 1.

26. Rusk Papers, Folder 287.

27. Rusk Papers, Folder 288, p. 3.

28. Rusk Papers, Folder 290, pp. 2–8. The materials list scholarships supported by AKF.

29. Rusk Papers, Folder 288, p. 10.

30. A Swedish surgeon named Stenstrom appears frequently in the Korean historiography, affiliated with a hospital ship maintained at Pusan during the war. Specifically, Stenstrom is cited by Dr. Jae-Duk Lew of Yonsei University.

31. Reportedly it is also popular for couples to get surgery together.

32. Rusk Papers, Folder 289, p. 1.

33. Khoo, "Some Aspects of Plastic (Cosmetic) Surgery in Orientals," pp. 60–69.

34. Millard, *Cleft Craft*.

35. Klein, *Cold War Orientalism*. For the Korean context, the Howard Rusk Papers contain many such images.

36. Shirakabe et al., "The Double-Eyelid Operation in Japan," pp. 224–241.

37. *Ibid.*

38. Gilman, *Making the Body Beautiful*, pp. 98–111.

39. *Ibid.*,p. 100.

40. There is a growing literature in the Korean visual arts tradition illustrating changing conceptions of beauty (and specifically in the eye area).

41. This is a speculative point, given the frequency of intersection between the two communities, as in Fruhstuck's *Colonizing Sex*.

42. Baek et al., "Oriental Blepharoplasty: Single-Stitch, Nonincision Technique," pp. 236–242. See especially p. 241.

43. Sayoc, "Plastic Construction of the Superior Palpebral Fold."

44. Khoo, "Some Aspects of Plastic (Cosmetic) Surgery in Orientals," pp. 60–69.

45. *Ibid.*

46. Haiken, *Venus Envy*. See chapter 5 in particular, "The Michael Jackson Factor: Race, Ethnicity, and Cosmetic Surgery."

47. *Ibid.*, pp. 199–201.

48. *Ibid.*, p. 201.

49. Wilson, "Medical Tourism in Thailand," p. 128.

50. This story appears in Haiken's chapter 5.

51. Shirakabe et al., "The Double-Eyelid Operation in Japan," p. 234.

52. *Ibid.* See Fernandez, "Double Eyelid Operation in the Oriental in Hawaii," pp. 257–264.

53. Kim and Jae-Duk Lew, "Clinical Study of Side-Effect Following the Injection of Foreign Substance in Cosmetic Plastic Surgery." This is one of the earliest abstracts referencing the subject explicitly, indicating that a great deal of undocumented activity was also taking place.

54. This trend continues today, with many clinics benefiting from the failures of their competitors.

55. *Songbaek Yu Chae-dŏk Kyosu Hwagap Kinyŏm Nonmun Mongnokchip. Yŏnse Taehakkyo Ŭigwa Taehak Sŏnghyŏng Oegwahak Kyosil p'yŏn (Collected research papers of Professor Jae-Duk Lew and his co-workers.)*

56. Again, the date here has to remain somewhat flexible, but given the appearance of abstracts such as the one in note 53, we can assume that it is roughly accurate.

57. This chronology is taken from the introductory section to the *Korean Society of Plastic and Reconstructive Surgery* memorial volume available at SNUH. It is also possible to locate abstracts for professional meetings from this time. See *Plastic and Reconstructive Surgery*, April 1969, for a brief summary of the Korean Society of Plastic and Reconstructive Surgery Meeting held November 8, 1968.

58. *Songbaek Yu Chae-dŏk Kyosu Hwagap Kinyŏm Nonmun Mongnokchip.*

59. *Ibid.*

60. Wolfort and Kanter, *Aesthetic Blepharoplasty*, p. 143.

61. Korean practitioners now frequently combine blepharoplasty and ecinathoplasty, giving them a reputation for favoring a radical, invasive style of surgery.

62. Chen, *Asian Blepharoplasty: A Surgical Atlas.*

63. *Ibid.*

64. *Ibid.*

65. *Ibid.*

66. Baek et al., "Oriental Blepharoplasty: Single-Stitch, Nonincision Technique," pp. 236–242. See also Bang, "The Double Eyelid Operation without Supratarsal Fixation," pp. 12–17.

67. Baek et al., "Oriental Blepharoplasty: Single-Stitch, Nonincision Technique."

68. *Ibid.*, p. 241.

69. *Ibid.*

70. See *Sŏnghyŏng oekwa ui ipchi wa pangmun yoin e kwanhan yŏn'gu.*

71. Lee, "The Politics of National Health Insurance in South Korea, 1961–1989." By the same author, see also "Health Care Reform in South Korea: Success or Failure?" pp. 48–51.

72. This does not mean that there were no payments involved, but many items provided were heavily subsidized.

73. So Yeon Leem of Seoul National University is currently working on a dissertation on the skin clinic in South Korea and has interviewed many of the major advocates of private care. So Yeon Leem, personal communication.

74. Also, this work would have been framed more typically within the field of ophthalmology.

75. Lee, "Health Care Reform in South Korea"; see section titled, "National Medical Insurance in Korea."

76. *Ibid.* The ROK government provides coverage in theory, but waiting for payment frustrates many doctors, encouraging them to move toward privatization.

77. Woo, *The Politics of Social Welfare Policy in South Korea*, p. 1.

78. Ma, "Medicine in the Making of Post-Colonial Korea."

79. This generalization is based on the first issues of the official journals associated with the respective societies as accessed at SNUH.

80. "Korea's New Face of Plastic Surgery."

81. *Ibid.*

82. *Ibid.*

83. See So-Yeon Leem's forthcoming dissertation.

84. I mean here a strengthening of the association between surgery and economic gain.

85. "IMF" would take on a range of meanings in the Korean context, such as "I Am Fired."

86. Kangnam Yonbo.

87. *Ibid.*

88. Kaw, "Medicalization of Racial features," pp. 74–89.

89. Millard, "Oriental Peregrinations."

90. This claim is made by the BK Dongyang clinic.

91. Uchida, "A Surgical Procedure for Blepharoptosis Vera and for Pseudo-Blepharoptosis Orientalis."

92. Donyang Clinic; available at http://english.bkdy.co.kr/resource/eyes.asp.

93. McCurdy and Lam, *Cosmetic Surgery of the Asian Face*. See chapter 2, "Asian Blepharoplasty," specifically the section titled "Upper Blepharoplasy."

94. *If You Were Me*, 2.

95. Lee, *Good for Her*.

Conclusion

1. Dr. Choo Kun Won, interview.

2. Park, *Jejoongwon*.

3. This slogan appears on the Yonsei campus and in the university's publicity materials.

4. See the Seoul National University fiftieth anniversary volume (*50-yŏnsa*) for the university's own account.

5. Morris-Suzuki, *Borderline Japan*, p. 94. To give a context, Morris-Suzuki is considering here the issue of ethnic Koreans remaining in Japan as of 1950; still, her figures suggest that many identified with "Chosŏn" rather than the new South Korea. Later, some of these individuals would repatriate to North Korea, a story told in Morris-Suzuki's *Exodus to North Korea*.

6. Brazinsky, *Nation-Building in South Korea*.

7. Brazinsky, "From Pupil to Model."

8. *The National Medical Center in Korea*, p. 32.

9. *Ibid.*

10. *Ibid.* See Appendix II, beginning from p. 89.

11. *Ibid.*

12. Park Bum-Soon of KAIST presented on this topic at ISHEASTM in 2008 (unpublished).

13. *Kŏn'gang*, August 1973, pp. 12–15.

14. There were small costs for most of these programs, but the objects (birth control, medications) were priced to meet the local market.

15. Au, *Mixed Medicines.*

16. Kim Seong-Jun, personal communication.

17. The *Yŏnbo* (annual reports) issued now by the government for the city of Seoul still list undocumented practitioners, emphasizing that this concern is considered a problem.

Bibliography

List of Archives and Collections Consulted

Harry S. Truman Presidential Library, Independence, MO (HST)
Korea Association for Health Promotion (KAHP), & Museum
Korea University (KU)
Kyunghee University (KYU)
National Archives II, College Park, MD (NARA)
National Diet Library, Tokyo, Japan (NDL)
National Library of Korea
National Archives of Korea
National Medical Center, Seoul, and Museum (NMC)
New York Public Library
New York University, Bobst Library
Princeton University, Mudd Manuscript Library, Princeton, NJ
Rockefeller Archive Center, Tarrytown, NY (RAC)
Seoul National University (SNU)
Seoul National University Hospital (SNUH)
Department of Parasitology and Tropical Medicine, Seoul National University
State University of New York (SUNY)-Buffalo
University of Michigan, Bentley Library, Ann Arbor, MI
University of Minnesota, Minneapolis, MN (UMN)
University of Missouri, Columbia, MO, Western Historical Manuscripts Collection (WHMC)
University of Virginia, Charlottesville, VA (UVA)
Yale University, Sterling Memorial Library, New Haven, CT (ST)
Yonsei University, Seoul, ROK (YUL)

Archival, Manuscript Collections

Charles Edward Amory Winslow Papers, Sterling Memorial Library, Yale University.

Byun Family Papers, in the possession of Dr. Byun Kil-won, accessed June 2006.

Records of the Army Specialized Training Division, Yale University, 1940–1963. See Accession 19ND-A-172. Civilian Affairs Training School. ST.

Records of the NYU Medical Center, 1942–1979. Bobst Library, University Archives, New York University.

Records of the School of Military Government, 1943–1945. U.S. Army School of Military Government, Special Collections. UVA.

Doctoral and Master's Theses (English and Korean)

Andrews, Bridie, J. "The Making of Modern Chinese Medicine, 1895–1937." DPhil, Cambridge University, 1996.

DeWall, Richard, "The Helix Reservoir Bubble Oxygenator for Use in Open Intracardiac Surgery." PhD dissertation, University of Minnesota, 1957.

Kim, Chong Bum. "Christianity in Colonial Korea: The Culture and Politics of Proselytization." PhD dissertation, Harvard University, 2004.

Kim Geun-Bae. "The Growth of Scientific-Technological Manpower during the Japanese Colonial Period." PhD thesis, Seoul National University, 1996.

Kim, Hoi-Eun. "Physicians on the Move: German Doctors in Meiji Japan and Japanese Medical Students in Imperial Germany, 1868–1914." PhD dissertation, Harvard University, 2006.

Kim, Jennifer Jung. "Gender and Modernity in Colonial Korea." PhD dissertation, UCLA, 2005.

Kim, Jongyoung. "Hybrid Modernity: The Scientific Construction of Korean Medicine in a Global Age." PhD dissertation, University of Illinois—Urbana Champaign, 2005.

Kim, Sonja M. "Contesting Bodies: Managing Population, Birthing, and Medicine in Korea, 1876–1945." PhD dissertation, UCLA, 2008.

Lee Chan-Bum. "Resection Therapy in Pulmonary Tuberculosis," M.S. thesis, Seoul National University, 1955.

Lee Hwang-Jun. "Minesot'a P'ŭrojekt'ŭ ka Han'guk Ŭihak Kyoyuk e Mich'in Yŏnghyang (The Influence of the Minnesota Project on Korean Medical Education)," PhD thesis, Seoul National University, 2006.

Lee, Jong-Chan, "The Politics of National Health Insurance in South Korea, 1961–1989." PhD dissertation. Johns Hopkins University, 1993.

Leem, Soyeon. "A Network of Things, Bodies, and Knowledge in Plastic Surgery Practice." PhD dissertation, Seoul National University, 2012.

Ma, EunJeong. "Medicine in the Making of Post-Colonial Korea, 1948 -2006." PhD dissertation, Cornell University, 2008.

Oh, Arissa Hyun Jung. "Into the Arms of America: The Korean Roots of International Adoption," PhD dissertation, University of Chicago, 2008.

Pae Ŭn-gyŏng, Han'guk Sahoe Ch'ulsan Chojŏl ŭi Yŏksajŏk Kwajŏng kwa Chendŏ: 1970–yŏndae Kkaji ŭi Kyŏnghŏm ŭl Chungsim ŭro (A Social history of Korean women's birth control: 1950s–1970s). Seoul: Seoul National University, 2003.

Park, Jinkyung. "Corporeal Colonialism: Medicine, Reproduction, and Race in Colonial Korea." PhD dissertation, University of Illinois at Urbana-Champaign, 2008.

Robertson (Suh), Jin Kyu. "Legacy of Empire: Japanese Influence on the United States Military Government in Korea in 1945." PhD dissertation, Harvard University, 2006.

Sawada, Chiho. "Cultural Politics in Imperial Japan and Colonial Korea: Reinventing Assimilation and Education Policy: 1919–1922." PhD dissertation, Harvard University, 2003.

Shin, Dong-Won. *Kungnip Ŭiwŏn Chejungwŏn,* 1885–1894. PhD dissertation, Seoul National University, 1995.

Smith, Hilary. "To Revise and to Improve: Historical Narrative in Traditional Chinese Medicine Textbooks in the PRC." MPhil thesis, Cambridge University, 2000.

Suh, Soyoung. "Korean Medicine between the Local and the Universal, 1600–1945." PhD dissertation, UCLA, 2006.

Taylor, Kim. "The History of the Barefoot Doctors." MPhil, Cambridge University, 1994.

———. "Medicine of Revolution: Chinese Medicine in Early Communist China (1945–1963)." DPhil thesis, Cambridge University, 2000.

Film

If You Were Me, 2. Korean Human Rights Commission, 2004.

Lee, Elizabeth. *Good for Her.* Los Angeles: Good for Her Productions, 2004.

Let's Live Well!/ "Chal sara pose!" [Mission Sex Control], 2006.

Interviews and Oral Histories

Dr. John Arnold, interview, UMN, November 2005. White Bear Lake, Minnesota.

Dr. Byun Kil-Won, interviews, June 16 and 25, 2006. Byun Family Clinic.

Dr. Choo Kun Won, interview, October 20, 2005, SNU Hospital, Alumni Building. The tape of the interview is in the possession of Dr. Kim Ock-Joo. SNUH.

Dr. Chu Jeong-hwa, interview, October 2, 2005. KUH.

Dr. Hong Sung-Tae, interviews, July and December 2010. SNUH.

National Medical Center Museum staff members, interviews, December 2010. NMC.

Crawford Sams. Oral history interview at WUSTL (re 1945–1951), retrieved on September 12, 2011 from http://beckerexhibits.wustl.edu/oral/transcripts/sams.html.

Horace G. Underwood, interviews, January 10 and 13 and February 13, 2003, conducted by e-mail.

Magazines, Published Materials

(English)

The Journal of Comparative Technology Transfer (Johns Hopkins University Press).

(Korean)

Chayu Segye [Free World], published by United States Information Service.

Kŏn'gang (Health). Seoul: KAPE, August 1973–.

Kŏn'gang Sosik (Health News). Seoul: KAPE, 1977–.

Taehak Sinmun (University News) (Seoul National University), 1950–1954

Personal Communication

Kim, Seong-Jun, Seoul National University, personal communication. May 2005,

Dr. Kim Tae-ho, SNUH, personal communication. February 2012,

Dr. Kim Won-Gon, SNUH, personal communication. August 2006.

Leem So-Yeon, SNU, personal communication. August 2010.

Pavel Leshakov, Moscow State University, May 2011, personal communication.

Primary Documents, Sources

(English)

Activities of Severance Union Medical College and Severance Hospital, 1927–28. Seoul: Severance Union Medical College. YUL.

"Background: Need for an Action Plan," in "Health and Social Affairs, Korea, Ministry of, 1962–1966." Box 26/FC, Population Council Accession #2. RAC.

Brown, E. P. "Report of Observation and Activities as Adviser in Medicine," January 24, 1959. UMN.

Certificate of voluntary status for Paul Hartman, "Equipment, 1964–1966," Box 26/ FC, Population Council, Accession #2, RAC.

Diehl, Dean H. S., Letter to Dr. George Schimert, January 27, 1958. Surgery Department 1007:33 "Schimert." UMN.

"Family Planning and Workers Creed," in PC FC #61, Population Council, Accession #2. RAC.

Flink, Edmund B. "Report and Recommendations on Teaching and Research in Internal Medicine," February 1, 1958. UMN.

Hartman, Paul. "Korea: Medical Referral System and Mobile Services." *Studies in Family Planning*, August 1966.

"Heart Refrigeration Operation—Lewis." Collection 875, Box 62. UMN.

History of Evacuation and Repatriation through the Port of Pusan, Korea, September 28, 1945–November 15, 1945.

"How to Insert an Intrauterine Loop," in "Taiwan, PSC, 1965–1966," Box 49, Population Council Accession, #2. RAC.

Kirk, Dudley. Letter of November 30, 1961, to John Y. Takeshita, Box PC / FC 50, Population Council Accession #2, RAC.

"Korea, Family Planning Program—Historical Review," in "Paul Hartman, 1967–1968," Box 26/FC, Population Council, Accession #2, RAC.

Lee Young-Gyun, Personal Papers & Surgical Records, in the possession of Dr. Kim Won-Gon, SNUH.

———. Letter of February 27, 1959. UMN.

———. Letter of August 24, 1959, UMN.

———. Letter of June 8, 1961, to W. Lillehei. UMN.

———. Letter of July 22, 1961, to W. Lillehei, UMN.

———. Letter of May 14, 1963, to W. Lillehei. UMN.

———. Letter of July 1, 1963, to W. Lillehei. UMN.

———. Letter of August 30, 1965, to W. Lillehei. UMN.

———. Letter of July 2, 1968, to W. Lillehei. UMN.

Stig Ljunggren, letter to Raymond Belsky, Box #47/FC, Population Council, Accession #2, RAC.

Maloney, William. "Report of Observations as Adviser in Medicine," July 1, 1956. UMN.

"Loop Production Problem." Box 25/FC, Population Council, Accession, #2. RAC.

Matthews, James H. "Final Report of Observations and Recommendations," November 7, 1958. UMN.

"Medical Conditions in Korea." Population Council, Accession #2, Box 25/FC, p. 1. RAC.

Minneapolis VA (Veterans Administration) Hospital. *Manual of Standard Procedures, Surgical Services*, pp. 2–9. 1007: 33, Surgery Department, VA Hospital 1955–1959. UMN.

Mitchell, Glenn R. "Report on the Seoul National University Hospital." UMN.

"Mobile Service, 1966." February 1967, Box PC FC #61, Population Council, Accession #2. RAC.

Monthly Summary of Nonmilitary Activities in Korea and Japan (SCAP/Supreme Command Allied Power), March 1947, "Student Unrest," p. 65. NARA II.

"Mr. Hill and Loop Experts." S. M. Keeney, 1964–1966, Box 26, FC, Population Council Accession #2, p. 1. RAC.

"Operation of Mobile Clinics Big Success." Annual Report of the Executive Officer, 1958–1959, p. 8, AKF (American-Korean Foundation), WHMC.

Organization of Family Planning Services, Korea. Box 26 / FC, Population Council, Accession #2, RAC.

"Organizational Report, April 1961-June 1963," PPFK, Box 26 / FC, Population Council, Accession #2, RAC, p. 1.

OTCA (Overseas Technical Cooperation Agency). Annual reports for the years 1966–1970. Tokyo: NDL.

"Paul P. Hartman, 1911–1968." Population Council, Accession, #2, Box PC FC #64, RAC.

PPFK (Planned Parenthood Foundation of Korea). *The 10-Year History of Family Planning in Korea*. Seoul: The Planned Parenthood Federation of Korea, 1976.

"Possible Employment of Mr. Paul Hartman as a Health Educator for Assignment to Korea." RAC.

"Preliminary Report of the Joint Kyunggi-Yonsei Family Planning Project (April 1968–March 1970)," in Folder "Jae Mo Yang," Box 27 FC, Population Council Accession #2. RAC.

Report of the Special Committee of the Faculty of Chosen Christian College," 378.51 C45e, Yonsei University, Rare Books and Special Collections.

Howard A. Rusk Papers. Folder 287, "American-Korean Foundation." WHMC.

———. Folder 288, "Report of Rusk Mission to Korea" (March 11–18, 1953). WHMC.

———. Folder 290, "Report to the President, Republic of Korea, by American-Korean Foundation, Second Mission." WHMC.

Schimert, George. Curriculum Vitae. SUNY Buffalo, University Archives.

———. *Final Report of Observations, Activities, and Recommendations Concerning the College of Medicine, Seoul National University*. October 7, 1959. UMN.

Severance Union Medical College Catalog, 1925–1926, 378.51 Se 83, p. 20. Rare Books and Special Collections, Yonsei University.

Keeny, S. M. Letter to Paul Hartman, November 25, 1965, in S. M. Keeny, Box 26/FC, Population Council, Accession #2. RAC.

Smith Report, "Some Problems in Public Health in Korea." Military Government Organization—Korea (Historical Summation); Report on Public Health Problems of South Korea (Draft Proposal ECA Program—Korea), Brig. Gen. Smith, USPHS, 1945–1953/File Unit from Record Group 331: Records of Allied Operational and Occupation Headquarters, World War II, Supreme Commander for the Allied Powers. Medical Section. Public Health and Welfare Division. Administration Section.

Staley, W. W. "Report on the College of Engineering, Seoul National University," August 1957, Lloyd Short Papers, Box 18, July–October 1957, UMN.

"Steps in Inserting the Lippes Loop." PC FC #61, Population Council, Accession #2. RAC.

"Summary of Field Observation of Kyunggi-Yonsei Family Planning Project." Population Council Accession #2, 27/FC. RAC.

"Sungdong Project." Box 26/FC, Population Council, Accession #2. RAC.

"Sung-dong Project: Key People." Population Council Accession #2, 26/FC. RAC.

"Sung-dong Project Substations," Population Council Accession #2, 26/FC. RAC.

Sung, Hee Yun. "Evaluation of Population Education Program for Young Male Adults: Knowledge and Interest Gain of Army Soldiers from Self-Instructional Learning Experience in the Republic of Korea." Box PC AD 52, Population Council, Accession #2. RAC.

Surgery Department 1007:33 "Schimert," UMN (Medical Faculty File for Schimert).

"Swedish Development Assistance in the Field of Family Planning, 1969," SIDA, Box AD 10 (Organizations), Population Council, Accession #2, RAC.

"Swedish Grant to Family Planning Programme of the Republic of Korea." Box 26 FC, Population Council Accession #2. RAC.

Tachi, Minoru. Letter of August 26, 1963, to Marshall Balfour, Folder Yang, Jae-Mo, Box 27/FC, Population Council, Accession #2. RAC.

"Training of Personnel." Box 27/FC, Population Council, Accession #2. RAC.

"Typhus, Small Pox Control Health Bureau's Big Task." RG 554, Box 20, "Public Health & Welfare, Health of Troops."

"TV spot announcement (radio spot announcement and newspaper ad)." Box 26/FC, Population Council accession #2, RAC.

Underwood, Horace H. "Education in Korea: The Situation and Some of the Problems," Report to SKIG (South Korean Interim Government), August 28t, 1947, p. 3. File 14.160, YUL.

The Veterans Administration Hospital and The University of Minnesota Medical School (pamphlet), 1007: 33 Surgery Department, VA Hospital, 1960–1961, UMN.

Wangensteen, Owen. Letter to George Schimert, February 3, 1958. Surgery Department 1007:33 "Schimert." UMN.

———. Letter to Dr. John Paine, April 27, 1960, p. 2. "Schimert." UMN.

———. "Report to Dean Howard's Subcommittee" (1965). UMN.

William Weems, letter of April 3, 1955 to James Morrill, President's papers, Collection 841, Box 107, "Foreign Operations Administration, September 1954–September 1955. UMN.

(Korean)

"Chubu ka toemyŏn nuguna" and "namp'yŏn i toemyŏn nuguna" ("Every housewife would like to/Every husband would like to"). PPFK, Box 26/FC, Population Council Accession #2, RAC.

Department of Parasitology and Tropical Medicine since 1954. Seoul: Seoul National University, 2004.

Kim Ock-Joo and Park Jiyoung, *Han'guk Singyŏng Oekwahak ŭi Sŏnguja*. Seoul: Seoul National University Press, 2011.

Kwon E. Hyock. *Kich'o Ŭihak kwa Ŭa ŭi Sam (Basic Medicine and My Life Are One/ United") 1923–*. Seoul: Sin'gwang Ch'ulp'ansa, 2009.

Licensing and Registration Certificate, 1947, Byun family papers, in the possession of Dr. Byun Kil-Won.

The Ordinances of the U.S. Military Government. Seoul Official Gazette, Choson haengjong ch'ulp'ansa, 1946.

PVC ŭi Kasoje. Anjŏngje e Kwanhan Yŏn'gu (PVC Research), KIST 1969 *Annual* 1969, p. 34.

Resumé /*iryŏksŏ* and Self-Introduction, 1947, Byun Family Papers.

Sŏul Taehakkyo Ŭigwahaksa Charyojip I {Seoul National University Medical History], SNUH.

Sŏnghyŏng Oegwa ŭi lipchi wa Pangmun Yoin e Kwanhan Yŏn'gu (Plastic Surgery Locations and Visits—A Study of Factors): Sŏul-si Kangnam-gu rŭl Chungsim ŭro/Yu, Chŏng-hwa, 1975. Parhaengsa: Sŏul Taehakkyo Taehagwŏn, 2003.

Vasectomy public health poster in the possession of Dr. Kim Nam-Il. KYU.

Secondary Works, Published: Academic Books, Articles, Newspapers

(English)

Aldous, Chris. "Typhus in Occupied Japan, an Epidemiological Study, 1945–1946," *Japanese Studies*, 26.3 (December 2006), pp. 317–333.

Aldous , Chris, and Suzuki, Akihito. *Reforming Public Health in Occupied Japan, 1945–1952: Alien Prescriptions?* London: Routledge, 2012.

Au, Sokhieng. *Mixed Medicines: Health and Culture in French Colonial Cambodia.* Chicago: University of Chicago Press, 2011.

Baek Se-Min et al. "Oriental Blepharoplasty: Single-Stitch, Nonincision Technique," *Plastic and Reconstructive Surgery*, 1989.

Baker, Don. "Oriental Medicine in Korea," in *Medicine across Cultures: History and Practice of Medicine in Non-Western Cultures*, Helaine Sellin, ed., pp. 133–154. Dordrecht, Boston, and London: Kluwer Academic Publishers, 2003.

Baldwin, Frank, Diane Jones, and Michael Jones. *America's Rented Troops: South Koreans in Vietnam.* Philadelphia: American Friends Service Committee, 1974.

Balfour, Marshall, Roger Evans, Frank Notestein, and Irene Taeuber. "Korea." *Public Health and Demography in the Far East.* New York: The Rockefeller Foundation, 1950.

Bang, Sook Man Gap Lee, and Jae Mo Yang. "A Survey of Fertility and Attitude toward Family Planning in Rural Korea." *Yonsei Medical Journal*, 4.1 (December 1963).

Bang, Yoo Hyun. "The Double Eyelid Operation without Supratarsal Fixation," *Plastic and Reconstructive Surgery*, 88.1 (July 1991), pp. 12–17.

Barry, John M. *The Great Influenza: The Story of the Deadliest Pandemic in History.* New York and London: Penguin Books, 2005.

"Birth Control Families to Get Apartment Priority," *The Korea Times*, April 27, 1975.

Brazinsky, Gregg. “From Pupil to Model: South Korea and American Development Policy during the Early Park Chung Hee Era,” *Diplomatic History*, 29.1 (January 2005), pp. 83–115.

———. *Nation-Building in South Korea: Koreans, Americans, and the Making of a Democracy.* Chapel Hill: University of North Carolina Press, 2007.

Bronfenbrenner, Martin. *Academic Encounter: the American University in Japan and Korea.* New York: Free Press of Glencoe, 1961.

Carafano, James. *Waltzing into the Cold War: The Struggle for Occupied Austria.* College Station: Texas A&M Press, 2002.

Chen, William Pai-Dei. *Asian Blepharoplasty: A Surgical Atlas.* Boston: Butterworth-Heinemann, 1995.

Cho Seung-Yull, “Parasitology in a Quickly Changing Society: Past Present and Future of Parsitology in Korea,” *The Korean Journal of Parasitology*, December 1990.

Clark, Donald. *Living Dangerously in Korea: The Western Experience, 1900–1950.* Norwalk, CT: Eastbridge, 2003.

Connelly, Matthew. *Fatal Misconception: The Struggle to Control World Population.* Cambridge, MA: Belknap Press of Harvard University Press, 2007.

“Conquest” Reports on Miraculous New Heart Surgery, March 9. CBS. UMN.

Cooper, David K. C. *Open Heart : The Radical Surgeons Who Revolutionized Medicine.* New York: Kaplan Publishing , 2010.

Cullather, Nick. *The Hungry World: America's Cold War Battle against Poverty in Asia.* Cambridge, MA: Harvard University Press, 2010.

Delaporte, Francis. *Disease and Civilization: The Cholera in Paris, 1832.* Cambridge, MA: MIT Press, 1986.

DiMoia, John. “Almatke Naasŏ Hullyunghage Kirŭja! (Let's Have the Proper Number of Children and Raise Them Well!)”: Family Planning and Nation-Building in South Korea, 1961–1968. *East Asian Science, Technology and Society: An International Journal*, 2.3 (2008).

———. “Atoms for Sale? Cold War Institution-Building and the South Korean Atomic Energy Project, 1945–1965,” *Technology and Culture*, 51.3 (July 2010), pp. 589–618.

Fernandez, Ramon. “Double Eyelid Operation in the Oriental in Hawaii,” *Plastic and Reconstructive Surgery Transplant Bulletin*, 25 (1960), pp. 257–264.

Freedman, Ronald. *Observing Taiwan's Demographic Transition: A Memoir*/Ronald Freeman. Published/Created: Taichung, Taiwan, ROC: Taiwan Provincial Institute of Family Planning; [Ann Arbor]: Population Studies Center, University of Michigan, 1998.

Freedman, Ronald and John Y. Takeshita, with contributions by L. P. Chow [and others]. *Family Planning in Taiwan: An Experiment in Social Change.* Princeton, NJ: Princeton University Press, 1969.

Frustuck, Sabine. *Colonizing Sex: Sexology and Social Control in Modern Japan.* Berkeley: University of California Press, 2003.

Gault , Neil. "Observations and Comments on the Seoul National University College of Medicine, Attached Hospital, School of Nursing, and School of Public Health, June 1961," pp. 80–81. UMN.

———. "Korea—A New Venture in International Medical Education." *University of Minnesota Medical Bulletin*, XXXIII (November 1961), pp. 73–85.

Gilles, Harold and D. R. Millard Jr. *The Principles and Art of Plastic Surgery*, 2 vols. Boston: Little, Brown, 1957

Gilman, Sander. *Making the Body Beautiful: A Cultural History of Aesthetic Surgery.* Princeton, NJ: Princeton University Press, 1999.

Gordin, Michael. *Five Days in August: How World War II Became a Nuclear War.* Princeton, NJ: Princeton University Press, 2007.

Grajdanzev, Andrew. *Modern Korea*. New York: International Secretariat, Institute of Pacific Relations, 1944.

Haiken, Elizabeth. *Venus Envy: A History of Cosmetic Surgery.* Baltimore, MD: Johns Hopkins University Press, 1997.

Han, Gil-Soo. "The Rise of Western Medicine and Revival of Traditional Medicine in Korea: A Brief History," *Korean Studies 21*, 1997: pp. 96–121.

Hartman, Paul. "Korea: Medical Referral System and Mobile Services," *Studies in Family Planning*, 13 (August 1966), pp. 10–12.

Henderson, Gregory. "Human Rights in South Korea, 1945–1953," in *Human Rights in Korea: Historical and Policy Perspectives*, William Shaw, ed. Cambridge, MA: Harvard University Press, 1991.

Holt, Bertha, with David Wisner. *The Seed from the East.* London: Oxford University Press, 1956.

Hong Sung-Tae et al. "A Successful Experience of Soil-Transmitted Helminth Control in the Republic of Korea." *Korean Journal of Parasitology*, 44.3 (September 2006), p. 178.

"How the U Helps Seoul University Rebuild after the Ravages of War." *The Minnesotan*, X.3 (December 1956).

Hughes, Carl. W. "Arterial Repair during the Korean War," *Annals of Surgery* (April 1958), pp. 555–561.

Hunter, G. W. III. "Local Health Hazards among US Troops Returning from Korea," *American Journal of Public Health*, November 1953, pp. 1408–1417.

Journal of Medical Education, December 1972, pp. 851–852.

Kato, K. *Introduction of a Thick Smear Technique with a Cellophane Cover for Helminth Eggs in Feces*. Pamphlet, Nagoya Public Medical Science Lab, 1968.

Kaw, Eugenia. "Medicalization of Racial Features: Asian American Women and Cosmetic Surgery," *Medical Anthropology Quarterly*, 7.1 (March 1993), pp. 74–89.

Khoo Boo-Chai, "Some Aspects of Plastic (Cosmetic) Surgery in Orientals," *British Journal of Plastic Surgery*, 22 (1969), pp. 60–69.

Kim, B. S., et al. "Parasitological Studies of Korean Forces in South Vietnam, II. A Comparative Study on the Incidences of Intestinal Parasites," *Korean Journal of Parasitology*, 8 (1970), p. 31.

Kim Byung Woo and Jae-Duk Lew, "Clinical Study of Side-Effect Following the Injection of Foreign Substance in Cosmetic Plastic Surgery," *New Medical Journal*, 15. 2 (1972).

Kim Dujong, *Han'guk Ŭihaksa (A History of Medicine in Korea)*. Seoul: Tamgudang, 1981.

———. "Middle Eastern and Western Influence on the Development of Korean Medicine," *Korea Journal* 2 (12) (1962): 5–7.

Kim, Eleana. *Adopted Territory: Transnational Korean Adoptees and the Politics of Belonging*. Durham, NC: Duke University Press, 2010.

Kim, Jin. "Chosŏn Sidae Ŭigwan Seonbal (Selection of Medical Officials during the Chosŏn Dynasty)" *Dongbang Hakchi* 104 (June 1999): pp. 1–93.

Kim, J. K. "A Socio-Medical Study in Vietnamese Rural Area," *Korean Journal of Public Health*, 1968, pp. 57–70.

Kim, Sonja. "In the Margins: Writing on Medicine in Korea after 1876," *Uisahak*, Dec. 2010), pp. 255–297.

———. "Limiting Birth: Birth Control in Colonial Korea, 1910–1945," EASTS, 2008 2 (3), pp. 335–359.

Klein, Christina. *Cold War Orientalism: Asia in the Middlebrow Imagination, 1945–1961*. Berkeley: University of California Press, 2003.

"Korea's New Face of Plastic Surgery," *Joongang Daily*, July 14, 2008. Retrieved in December 2010 from http://koreajoongangdaily.joinsmsn.com/news/article/article.aspx?aid=2892277.

Lada, John (ed.). Chapter XVI, "Philippines and Okinawa." in *Civil Affairs / Military Government Public Health Activities*, (*Preventive Medicine in World War II*, Volume VIII). Washington, DC: Office of the Surgeon General, Department of the Army, 1976.

———. Part V. The Pacific," in *United States in World War II, Medical Department*, United States Army, in *Preventive Medicine in World War II*, Volume VIII: Civil Affairs/Military Government, Public Health Activities, 1976.

Lankov, Andrei. *The Dawn of Modern Korea*. Seoul: EunHaeng NaMu Publishing, 2008.

Lee Byeong-cheon (ed.). *Developmental Dictatorship and the Park Chung-hee Era: The Shaping of Modernity in the Republic of Korea*. Seoul: Homa and Sekey, 2006.

Lee Hee Yong. "Studies on Vasectomy, 3: Clinical Studies on the Influences of Vasectomy." *Taehan Pinyo Kigwa Hakhoeji* (*The Korean Journal of Urology*).

Lee Jong-Chan. "Health Care Reform in South Korea: Success or Failure?"*American Journal of Public Health*. 93.1 (January 2003), pp. 48–51.

Lee, J. S., et al. "The Clinical Study of 157 Cases of Malaria Evacuated from Vietnam," *Journal of the Korean Medical Association*, 10, pp. 318–326.

Lee, S. H., et al. "Santonin-Kainic Acid Complex as a Mass Chemotherapeutic of Ascaris Lumbicoides Control in Korea," *Korean Journal of Parasitiology*, 10.2 (1972,), pp. 79–85.

Leeke, Ada. *When Americans Came to Korea*. Freeman, SD: Pine Hill Press, 1991.

Leem So Yeon and Jin Hee Park. "Rethinking Women and Their Bodies in the Age of Biotechnology: Feminist Commentaries on the Hwang Affair," *EASTS*, 2.1 (2008), pp. 9–26.

Lillehei, C. Walton, et al. "Direct Vision Intracardiac Surgery in Man Using a Simple, Disposable Artificial Oxygenator." *Diseases of the Chest*, 29 (1956), pp. 1–8.

Linker, Beth. *War's Waste: Rehabilitation in World War I America*. Chicago: University of Chicago Press, 2011.

McCurdy, John A., and Samuel Lam. *Cosmetic Surgery of the Asian Face*. New York: Thieme, 2005.

Meade, E. Grant. *American Military Government in Korea*. New York: King's Crown Press, 1951.

Millard, D. R. "Oriental Peregrinations," *Plastic and Reconstructive Surgery*, 16.5 (November 1955).

———. *Cleft Craft: The Evolution of Its Surgery*. Boston: Little, Brown, c1976–c1980.

———. *Saving Faces: A Plastic Surgeon's Remarkable Story*. Fort Lauderdale, FL: Write Stuff Syndicate, 2003.

Miller, Wayne. *King of Hearts: The True Story of the Maverick Who Pioneered Open Heart Surgery*. New York: Times Books, 2000.

Millett, Alan R. *The War for Korea, 1945–1950: A House Burning*. Lawrence: University Press of Kansas, 2005.

"A Modern Doctor Takes up a Traditional Business," *Joongang Daily*, January 27, 2006.

Moon, Seungsook. *Militarized Modernity and Gendered Citizenship in South Korea*. Durham, NC: Duke University Press, 2005.

Morris-Suzuki, Tessa. "'Invisible Immigrants': Undocumented Migration and Border Controls in Postwar Japan." *The Journal of Japanese Studies*, 32.1 (Winter 2006), pp. 119–153.

———. *Exodus to North Korea*. New York: Rowman & Littlefield, 2007.

———. *Borderline Japan: Foreigners and Frontier Controls in the Postwar Era*. Cambridge, UK, and New York: Cambridge University Press, 2010.

The National Medical Center in Korea: A Scandinavian Contribution to Medical Training and Health Development, 1958–1968. Oslo: Universitetsforlaget, 1971.

Palumbio-Liu, David. *Asian/American: Historical Crossings of a Racial Frontier.* Palo Alto, CA: Stanford University Press, 1999.

Rim, H. J. "The Incidence of Intestinal Parasites in ROK Army Soldiers," *Korean Journal of Parasitology*, 1963.

Rusk, Howard A. *A World to Care For: The Autobiography of Howard Rusk*. New York: Random House, 1972.

Sams, Crawford. *"Medic": The Mission of an American Military Doctor in Occupied Japan and Wartorn Korea*. New York and London: M. E. Sharpe, 1998.

Sayoc, B. T. "Plastic Construction of the Superior Palpebral Fold," *American Journal of Ophthalmology* 38 (1954).

Schmid, Andre. *Korea between Empires, 1885–1919*. New York: Columbia University Press, 2002.

Sellin, Helaine, ed. *Medicine across Cultures: History and Practice of Medicine in Non-Western Cultures*. Dordrecht, Boston, and London: Kluwer Academic Publishers, 2003.

Seo, B. S., and H. J. Rim. "A Study of Malaria amongst Narcotic Addicts in Seoul," *Seoul University Journal*, 8.

Seo, B. S., et al., "Parasitiological Studies of Korean Forces in South Vietnam, I. Examinations of Blood Films on Malaria Patients," *Korean Journal of Parasitology*, 8 (1970).

Shin Dong-Won. "The License System for Korean Herbal Practitioners in 1900," in *Current Perspectives in the History of Science in East Asia*, Yung Sik-Kim and Francesca Bray eds., pp. 478–483. Seoul: Seoul National University Press, 1999.

Shin Gi-Wook and Michael Robinson. *Colonial Modernity*. Cambridge, MA: Harvard University Asia Center, Harvard University Press, 1999.

Shirakabe, Yukio, et al. "The Double-Eyelid Operation in Japan: Its Evolution as Related to Cultural Changes," *Annals of Plastic Surgery*, 15.3 (September 1985), pp. 224–241.

Park Hyung Woo. *Jejoongwon: The First Westernized Hospital* in Korea. Seoul: Body and Mind Books, 2002.

Rogaski, Ruth. *Hygienic Modernity: Meanings of Health and Disease in Treaty-Port China*. Berkeley: University of California Press, 2004.

Rusk, Howard A. *A World to Care For: The Autobiography of Howard A. Rusk, M.D.* New York: Random House, 1972.

Schimert, George. "A Simple Bubble Type of Pump-Oxygenator for Intracardiac Surgery." *Surgery*, 40.6 (December 1956), pp. 1018–1022.

———. "A Review of the Present State of Intracardiac Surgery." *New Medical Journal*, 1.1 (1958), pp. 68–73.

Seoul through Pictures, Volume 4: Seoul, To Rise Again. Seoul: The City History Compilation Committee, 2005.

Seth, Michael. *Education Fever: Society, Politics and the Pursuit of Schooling in South Korea*. Honolulu: University of Hawaii Press, 2002.

Son, Annette, H. K. "Modernization of Medical Care in Korea, 1876–1990," *Social Science & Medicine* 49 (1999), pp. 543–550.

Takeshita, Chikako. *The Global Biopolitics of the IUD*. Cambridge, MA: MIT Press, 2011.

"They Appreciate Dogs That Died." *The Minneapolis Star*, October 15, 1952. UMN.

"Townspeople Send Girl, 3, Here for Surgery." *The Minneapolis Star*, February 3, 1958. UMN.

Turner, Thomas. "Chapter XVIII: Japan and Korea," in in *Civil Affairs / Military Government Public Health Activities*, (*Preventive Medicine in World War II*, Volume VIII), pp. 659–707. Washington, DC: Office of the Surgeon General, Department of the Army, 1976.

Uchida, Juinichi. "A Surgical Procedure for Blepharoptosis Vera and for Pseudo-Blepharoptosis Orientalis," *British Journal of Plastic Surgery*, 15 (1962), pp. 271–276.

Underwood, Elizabeth. *Challenged Identities: North American Missionaries in Korea, 1884–1934*, Seoul: Royal Asiatic Society, 2003.

Underwood, Horace. *Korea in War, Revolution and Peace: The Recollections of Horace G. Underwood*. Edited and Annotated by Michael J. Devine. Seoul: Yonsei University Press, 2001.

Wells, Ken. "The Rationale of Korean Economic Nationalism under Japanese Colonial Rule, 1922–1932: The Case of Cho Man-sik's Products Promotion Society," *Modern Asian Studies* 19, 4 (1985), pp. 822–859.

West, Patricia J., with Wilmer J. Coggins. *A Special Kind of Doctor: a History of the College of Community Health Sciences*. Tuscaloosa, AL: CCHS, 2004.

Willard, William R. "Some Problems in Public Health Administration in the U.S. Army Military Government in Korea." *Yale Journal of Biology and Medicine*, March 1947, pp. 661–670.

———. *Medical Education and Medical Care in Alabama: Some Inadequacies, Some Solutions*. Tuscaloosa, AL: College of Community Health Sciences, 1983.

Wilson, Ara. "Medical Tourism in Thailand," in *Asian Biotech*, Aiwha Ong and Nancy Chen, eds. Durham, NC: Duke University Press, 2010.

Wolfort, Francis, and William R. Kanter. *Aesthetic Blepharoplasty*. Boston: Little, Brown and Company, 1995.

Wong, Joseph. *Healthy Democracies: Welfare Politics in Taiwan and South Korea*. Ithaca, NY: Cornell University Press, 2004.

———. *Betting on Biotech: Innovation and the Limits of Asia's Develomental State*. Ithaca, NY: Cornell University Press, 2011.

Woo, Myungsook. *The Politics of Social Welfare Policy in South Korea: Growth and Citizenship*. Lanham, MD: University Press of America, 2004.

Yang, Daqing. *Technology of Empire: Telecommunications and Japanese Expansion in Asia, 1883–1945*. Cambridge, UK, and London: Harvard East Asia, 2010.

Yang Jae-Mo. "A Comprehensive Study of the Health Needs, Health Care, and Physicians' Income in Cheju Do," Yonsei Medical Journal, 1959.

———. "A Comprehensive Study of Health Needs and of Health Care in Seoul," *Yonsei Medical Journal*, 1.1 (December 1960), pp. 71–76.

(Korean)

Chi Je Geun. "Sŏul Taehakkyo Ŭigwa Taehak Pyŏngnihak Kyosil 50-yŏnsa (First 50 Years of Department of Pathology Seoul National/First 50 Years of Department of Pathology Seoul National University College of Medicine)," *Korean Journal of Medical History*, 5.1 (June 1996), pp. 33–52.

Department of Neurosurgery, Seoul National University College of Medicine: 50th Anniversary (1957–2007). Seoul, Korea : Academya Publishing Company, 2007.

Han'guk Haksaeng Hoech'ung Kamyŏm Chiptan Kwalli Saŏp Punsŏk: Hoech'ung 10-yŏnsa 1969–78 [Students survey, 10 years of anti-parasite]/Han'guk Kisaengch'ung Pangmyŏl Hyŏphoe p'yŏn. [Sŏul]: Han'guk Kisaengch'ung Pangmyŏl Hyŏphoe, 1980.

Kamsajang, in the possession of Dr. Byun Kil-won, Byun Family Papers.

Kangnam Statistical Yearbook, Seoul City Government, 2006.

Kim Ock-Joo and Hwang, Sang-ik. "The Minnesota Project: The Influence of American Medicine on the Development of Medical Education and Medical Research in Post-war Korea." *Korean Journal of Medical History* (June 2000), pp. 112–123.

Kisaengch'unghak Kyosil 50-yŏnsa [50 years parasitology], 2004.

Kwon E. Hyock. *Ten Years of Urban Population Studies in Korea*. Seoul: Seoul National University Press, 1974.

Moon Man-Young and Kim Young-Sik. *Han'guk Kŭndae Kwahak Hyŏngsŏng Kwajŏng Charyo (Documentary History of the Development of Modern Science in Korea)*. Seoul: Seoul National University Press, 2004.

Paeumyŏ Karŭch'imyŏ [Learning and Teaching], 40th annual volume, SNU Department of Parsitology and Tropical Medicine, 1994.

Park Hyung Woo et al. "Chaedong Chejungwŏn ŭi Kyumo wa Hwaktae Kwajŏng (A Study on the Location and Function of the Jaedong Jejoongwon)," *Korean Journal of Medical History*, June 2000, pp. 29–53.

Pictorial History of Modern Medicine in Korea. Seoul: Woongjin, 2009.

Prevalence of Intestinal Parasitic Infections in Korea, the 3rd and 4th reports, 1981, 1985 surveys, SNUH library.

Shin Dong-Won. *Hoyŏlcha, Chosŏn ŭl Sŭpkyŏk Hada [Cholera's attack on Choson]: Mom kwa Ŭihak ŭi Han'guksa*. Seoul: Yŏksa Pip'yŏngsa, 2004.

Shin Jwa Sup. "Kunjŏnggi ŭi Pogŏn Ŭiryo Chŏngch'aek" ("Policy of USAMGIK toward Public Health and Medicine in Occupied South Korea"), *Korean Journal of the History of Medicine*, 9.2 (December 2000), pp. 212–232.

Songbaek Yu Chae-dŏk Kyosu Hwagap Kinyŏm Nonmun Mongnokchip. Yŏnse Taehakkyo Ŭigwa Taehak Sŏnghyŏng Oegwahak Kyosil p'yŏn. (Collected research papers of Professor Jae-Duk Lew and his co-workers in commemoration of his sixtieth birthday), Sŏul: Yemun'gak, Yonsei University, January 9, 1990.

Sŏul Taehakkyo Hyungbu Oegwahak Kyosil (Seoul National University Thoracic Surgery). Seoul: National University Press, 2000.

The 30 Year History of Hyundai Construction. Seoul: 1977.

Yeo In-sok, "Han Mal kwa Ilche Sigi Sŏn'gyo Ŭisadŭl ŭi Chŏnt'ong Ŭihak Insik kwa Yŏn'gu (The Gaze of the Others: How the Western Medical Missionaries Viewed the Traditional Korean Medicine)." *Korean Journal Medical History*. June 2006: pp. 1–21.

Speeches, Public Addresses

Harry S. Truman, Inaugural Address (the "Point Four Speech"), January 20, 1949; Details of the Point Four program can be found at http://www.trumanlibrary.org/hstpaper/point4.htm.

Websites

BK Donyang Clinic / http://english.bkdy.co.kr/center/eyes/. Retrieved November 13, 2012.

Kaleida Health. Retrieve in June 2011 from www.kaleidahealth.org/news/archive/1200/121200.asp.

National Archives of Korea; retrieved on November 11, 2012, from www.koreanhistory.or.kr/.

Sigmamotor, Inc. Retrieved on Noverrmber 12, 2012, from http://sigmamotorinc.com/history_sigma_motor.html.

University of Minnesota, Department of Neurosurgery; retrieved on November 12, 2012, from http://www.neuro.umn.edu/History/peyton/home.html

Yonsei University College of Medicine, retrieved November 11, 2012, from http://medicine.yonsei.ac.kr/en/About_YUCM/Introduction.

Yonsei University Severance Hospital; retrieved on September 20, 2001, from www.yuhs.or.kr/en/hospitals/severance/clinic_dept/Pulmo_dept/intro/

Yonsei University Medical College; retrieved from http://yuhs.iseverance.com/en/about_yuhs/yuhs/YUMC_history/index.asp.

Index

Page numbers with fig. denote illustrations.

FSC
www.fsc.org
MIX
Papier | Fördert
gute Waldnutzung
FSC® C083411

Kolibri 360 GmbH
Ferdinand-Jühlke-Straße 7
99095 Erfurt, Deutschland
produktsicherheit@kolibri360.de